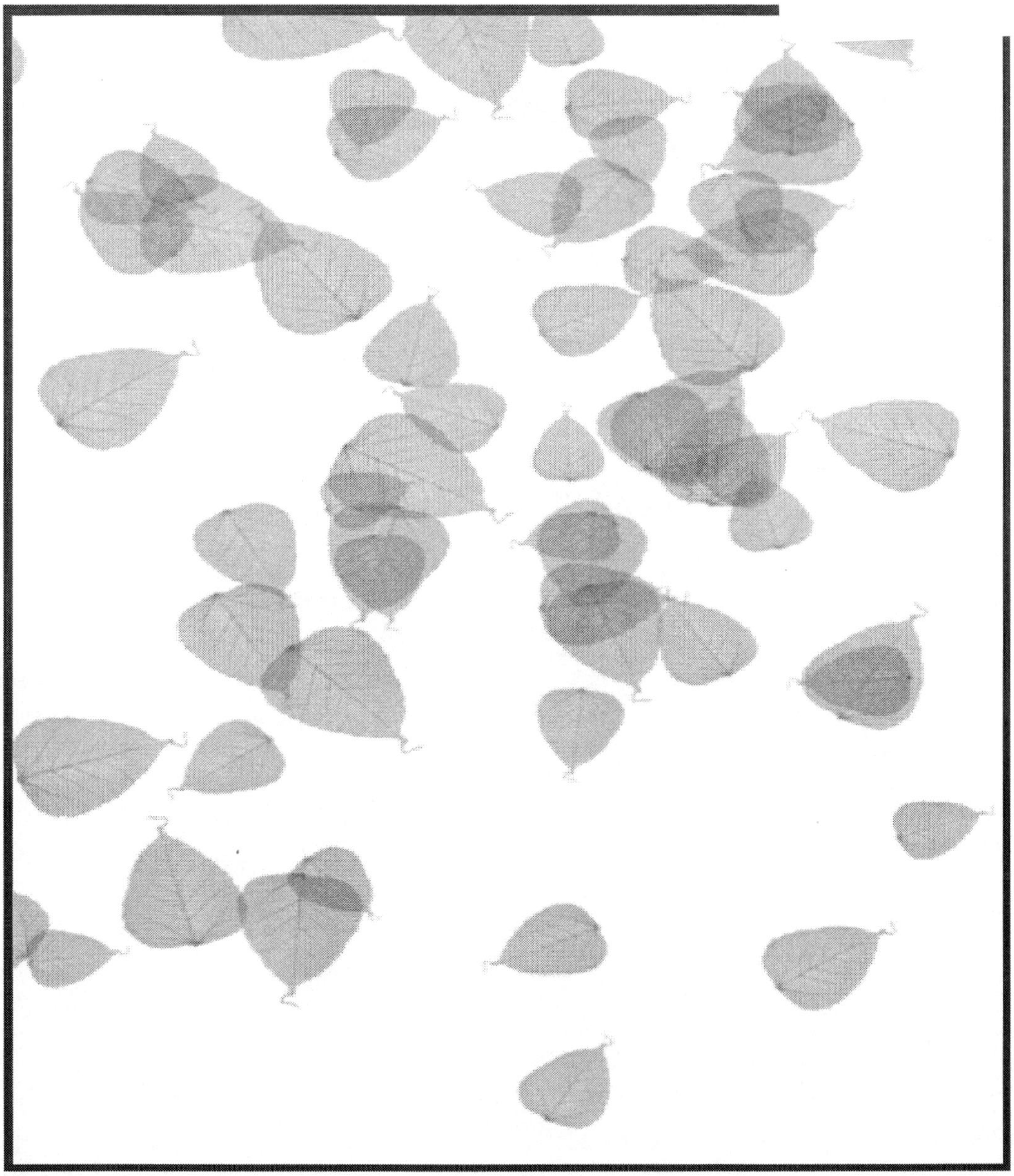

The Humble Beginning of an Immortal

Norm Than

The Humble Beginning of an Immortal

© Copyright 2006. By Norm Than.

Published by Lulu Enterprises
860 Aviation Parkway
Suite 300
Morrisville, NC 27560
United States

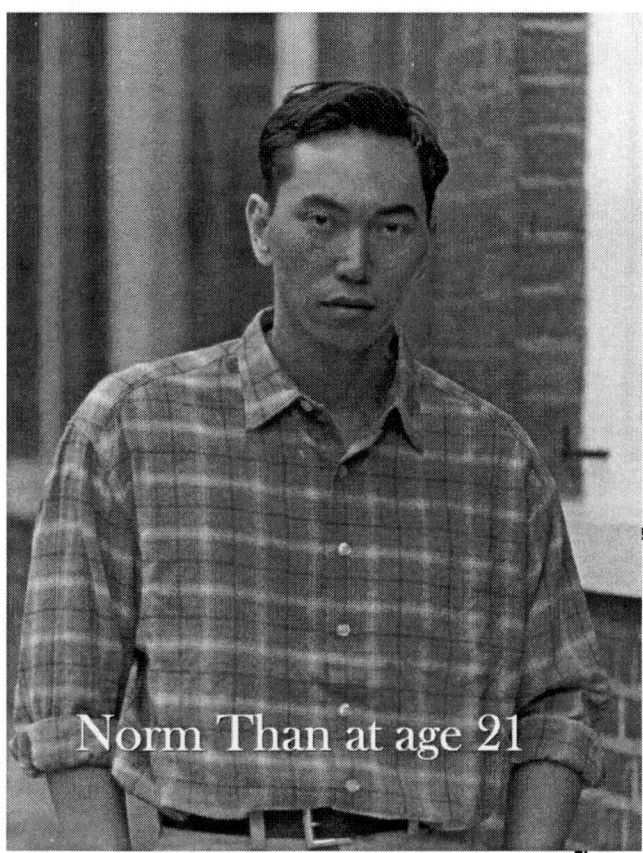

Norm Than at age 21

The seeds of immortality were planted at an early age. The ancient Chinese teachings of Taoism and its mystical practice of the Three Treasures were deeply rooted within

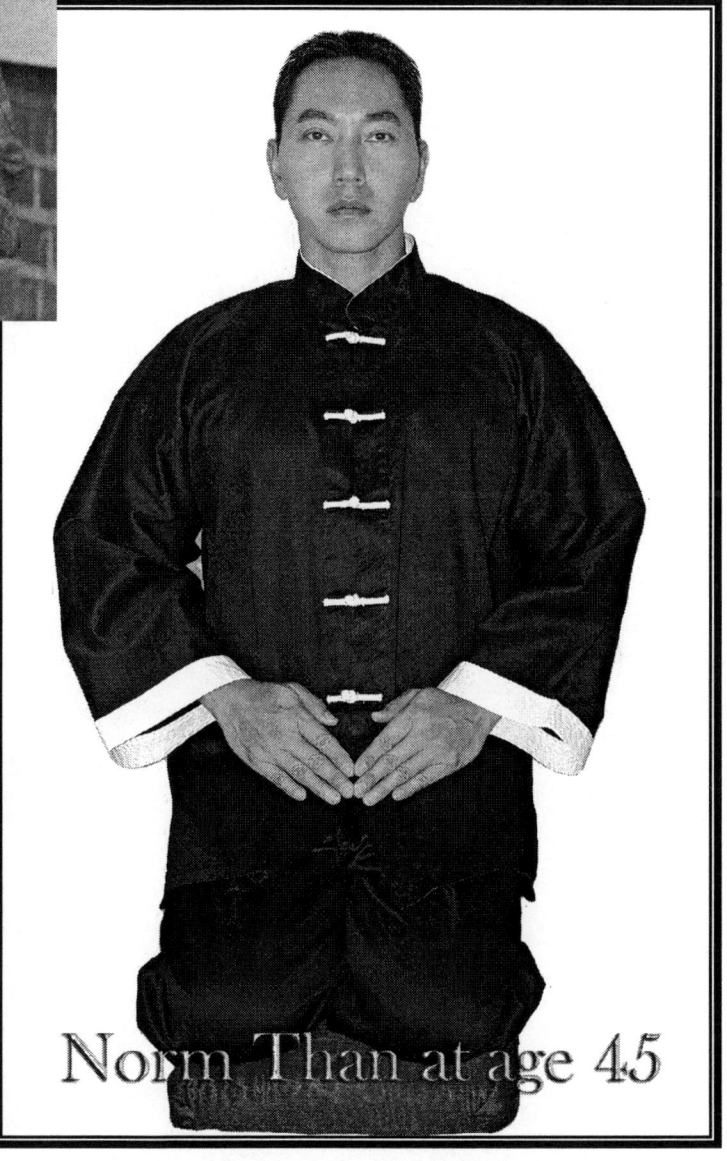

Norm Than at age 45

to guide and nurture this young man to uncover the primordial secrets of Youthful Immortality. His path of self-discovery uncovers shocking answers about himself and the destiny for humanity.

"Immortality is the final evolutionary step for all Humanity"

Qi Gong Master Norm Than

Contents

The Conception of Immortality

As a young boy I was fascinated with the idea of Immortality. I believed immortality was a gift from nature as the final stage of humanity's evolution. Today as a mature adult I still deem this concept to be true. Immortality remains humanity's greatest challenge and never ending quest. In our modern world the search for immortality still carries on with inventions of pills, rigorous diets and contraptions to prolong life. Medical technology has provided expensive drugs, medicine, plastic surgery and hormone therapy in the hopes of reaching immortality but these efforts are limited at best. Though the average lifespan has been extended, many are left to age in misery from health problems associated with advanced age. This is a far cry from the vision many have of living a prolonged life. I, so like many others, believe that immortality is one of remaining young, healthy and full of energy as we grow older, and have dedicated my life to achieving this.

I discovered at a young age that the answer to achieving immortality was not in the future but in our ancient past. Thousands of years ago, in ancient China the secret wisdom of immortality was practice by mystical hermits called Taoist sages. These ancient sages followed the path of Taoism and reportedly lived hundreds of years, some even achieved immortality. Taoism has its own version of the Fountain of Youth called Youthful Immortality. All Taoist sages inspired to be what is termed, a Youthful Immortal. A Youthful Immortal is one who has managed to obtain the secrets of life at a relatively young age, and as a result is able to remain younger and healthier than his grandchildren or great grandchildren.

One can only achieve this state of immortality when they have mastered the Three Treasures. The ancient sages held their own secret methods and forms to attaining Youthful Immortality but all adhered to preserving the Three Treasures. The first Treasure was the Ching (human body), the second was Qi (breath) and the third was Shen (spirit). It was thought that if one can develop and restore the Three Treasures, one would obtain Youthful Immortality.

I have dedicated my life to learning, practicing and mastering the Taoist Three Treasures, and believe I have taken the first steps on the sacred path to achieving Youthful Immortality.

My own self revelation came in two parts. The first part came when I discovered Taoism and the Three Treasures. The second part was when I finally discovered the 'True Master' of Qi and immortality. I spent a lifetime cultivating the Three Treasures and as a result I look about half my age and with that, set in motion my journey on the path to becoming a Youthful Immortal.

Youthful Immortality
– The Final Frontier

From his book, 'Ageless Body, Timeless Mind', author Deepak Chopra coined the phrase 'New' old age to represent the current health and fitness status of seniors. In the past, the phrase "Old' old age, would apply to people growing up during the depression and two world wars. When they reached retirement age they were old and feeble. Since the sixties and seventies, through medical technology and changing lifestyles, our current seniors are as active and fit as their younger counterparts, therefore forcing a change in the way we look at seniors and rephrasing "Old" old age to 'New' old age. But regardless of how full of life these 'New' old age seniors were, they still showed their age!

But today and future generations to come the final evolutionary stage of humanity has commenced with 'The Humble Beginning of an Immortal' The quest for the Fountain of Youth would finally be realized through the knowledge and practice of the ancient Taoist sages by one contemporary Youthful Immortal (and that's me!).

A Layman's Guide
to Immortality

The reason I have chosen to write this book is that unlike the ancient sages I believe Youthful Immortality may be obtained by ordinary people. One doesn't have to live as a hermit and or become a Taoist sage to achieve longevity (a long life). Immortality isn't only for Michael Jackson and his specialized O2 tank, it isn't just for the rich, educated, and religious or anyone who studied martial arts or TCM (Traditional

Chinese Medicine), it can be achieve by anyone who will adhere to the practice of the Three Treasures.

Since I believe that one does not need special knowledge to practice the Three Treasures to achieve longevity, I have written this book without the usual esoteric jargon, and limited the use of confusing terms and long-winded names so often seen in other books. I didn't write this book in a way to put myself above others. I wrote it in plain English, in a simple, easy to read and understand format as I wanted the books I read to be. As I was developing the Three Treasures I realized it was unnecessary to know or master everything regarding Taoist practices to achieve immortality. It was unnecessary to have an understanding of where and how all the channels and meridians (invisible pathways throughout the body) worked. It was unnecessary to be an expert in TCM (the ancient Taoist sages were the original practitioners of using herbs to cure illnesses). It was unnecessary to become a religious guru, or join a cult or twist your body into a knot and or change your first name to Swami.

'The Tao that can be described
is not the eternal Tao'

However, before one goes rushing in to practice my version of the Taoist Three Treasures, it is beneficial to have at least some understanding of Taoism.

So what is Taoism? Taoism is one of the oldest philosophical and religious traditions in the world. Taoism originated as a philosophy but quickly developed some religious aspects to it, in other words one can see it as a philosophy or a religion or both. The heart of Taoism is its system of living in balance with nature. Beneath this central idea is the wisdom of achieving a healthy and long life, even obtaining immortality. One reason the Taoist concept of immortality came about was because it was believed that it took one years to prepare the Shen (Spirit) for transformation and therefore a long life was needed.

Taoism has been practiced many years before it was ever given the name, which was around the Han dynasty (around 206 B.C. to 220 A.D.) Taoism expresses itself in awe of nature with a central theme of acceptance of nature. It views humans as part of nature and their actions are of natural spontaneity (path or guide of man) in accordance with nature.

The two most important figures in Taoism are Laozi and Zhuangzi. Laozi lived around the sixth century B.C. and is considered the 'founder of Taoism' and author of the Daode Jing. Zhuangzi arrived after Laozi (around third century B.C.) and is the author of Zhuangzi.

One thing to know when you start understanding Taoism is the term Tao. Tao may be translated as 'path' or 'way' or 'guide' It's the way things reliably work. There are little taos such as the tao of man, the tao of nature but there is only one big Tao or Great Tao (the Tao of the Universe). There is a famous Taoist scripture that literally reads 'a tao can tao not constant tao' but when translated it reads something like 'The tao that can be described is not the eternal tao' Huh? Not to worry! Here is a brief summary of what I believe is the hidden meaning behind this famous scripture. Taoism, that is Laozi and Zhuangzi, were skeptical of society's moral rules of conduct, language, laws and government etc. In other words, they were skeptical of what society thinks it knows is best, more specifically they were skeptical of society's knowledge. They believe that humans are limited with limited knowledge and the Great Tao is limitless. To spend ones limited lifetime to try and understand the limitless is a waste. We would never know everything so we can never be sure if what we are doing (morals of conduct) or saying (language) or our perspectives (judgments) are actually the correct ones! So when we say this or that about a certain tao or try to describe it we can't be certain it is right because it comes from a limited point of view and understanding!

Other Taoist stuff

In order to understand and possibly achieve Youthful Immortality, one should get acquainted with some basics terms I will use throughout this book. Ready? Here we go...

What is Qi? Qi is an invisible life energy that travels through meridians or channels (pathways throughout the body) to the entire body. What is Qi Gong? Qi Gong is a form of exercise consisting of slow movements created by Taoist sages to cultivate and transmit Qi. What is Yi? Translated Yi means something like Intention or Will. It is what the practitioner uses to move or transmit Qi. What is Wei Wu? Translated wei wu means 'Without doing' or lack of action. It doesn't mean being lazy but giving up pointless struggles but yet still managing to get things done. It also means responding authentically and spontaneously to circumstances in one's surrounding. What is Dantien or Dan Tien? It is the area just below the navel which is consider ones centre and where Qi is cultivated. What is Micro Cosmic Orbit? Also known as the Lesser Heavenly Circuit, it is the imaginary circuit that runs from the Dantien to the back of the tailbone, up the spine and neck to the head and is reconnected once the tongue is placed on the roof of the mouth, and back down the front of the chest to the Dantien again. The more Qi that runs through the Micro Cosmic Orbit the better ones chances of obtaining health and longevity.

OK, that should be enough for now. Don't worry if you still don't understand some of the terminology, I'll be repeating them throughout the book. The main purpose is just to get an idea behind Taoist Immortality.

My brother Eddie

I would like to dedicate this book to my family and especially to my big brother Eddie. His love, encouragement, support and understanding has made this book possible. As the youngest in my family I have always looked up to my big brother. My brother Eddie is kind, generous, royal and forgiving. To me, Eddie represented the type of person I wanted to be like when I grew up. He has been my guide and inspiration from childhood and still is today. My love for him has no bounds or limitations.

'Thanks Eddie, for everything!'

From your little brother, Norm

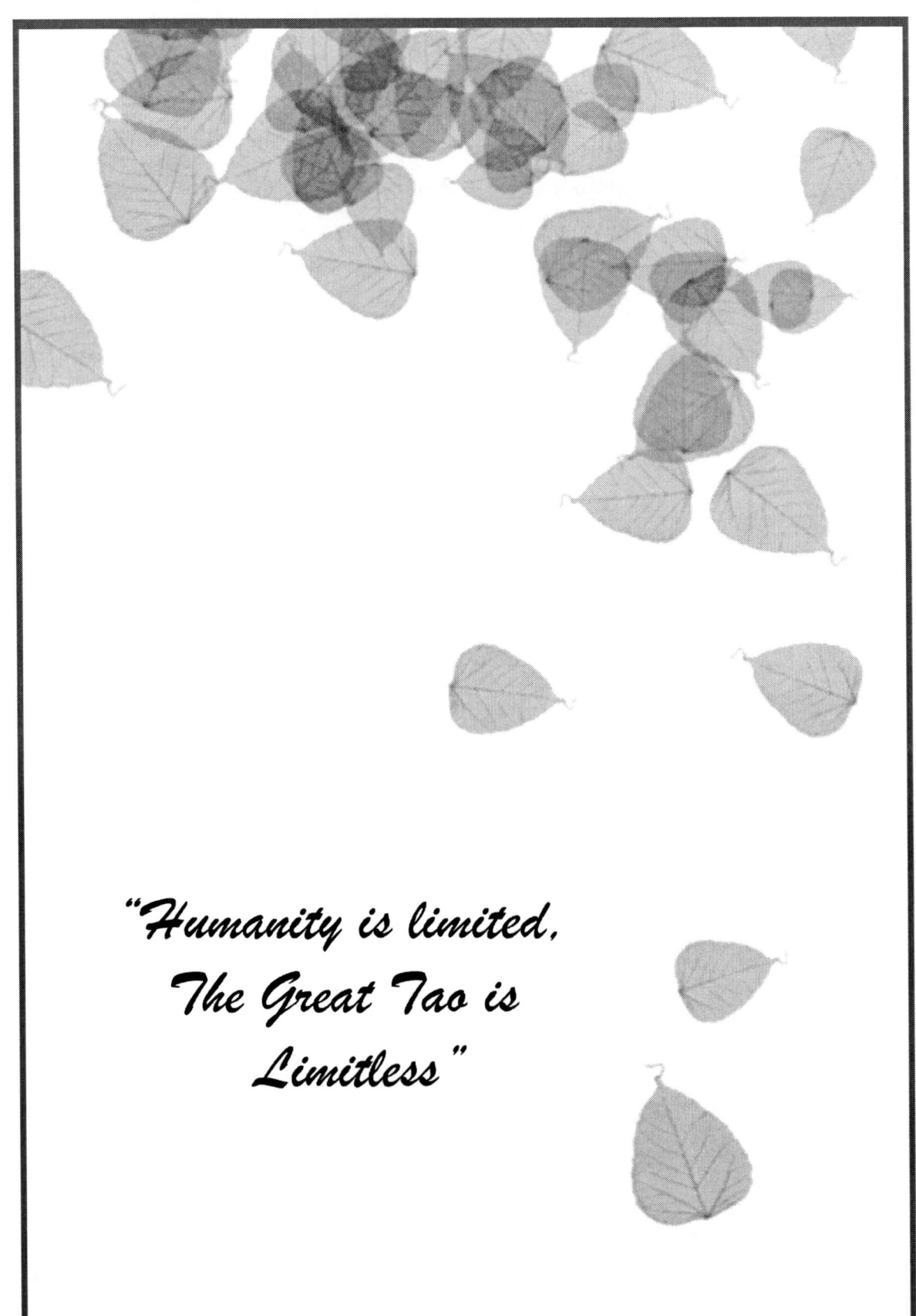

"Humanity is limited,
The Great Tao is
Limitless"

The Tao of the Norm

Introduction

In obtaining Youthful Immortality, a lifetime of commitment was required of me! The journey was both arduous and laborious with infinite rewards.

But the most challenging part was actually writing about my maiden voyage into the unknown realms of eternal life. Surpassing the barriers of old age while resetting the evolutionary standards of humanity is not an everyday occurrence. So how do I even begin to explain such an event? How do I jot down a lifetime of analyzing, observing, experimenting and training? It is a task of mammoth portions yet, as introvert and personal as I am, I find within myself an overwhelming intrinsic need to record my life story.

Everyone's favorite book is always the one written about them; and my book is no exception to that rule. The most difficult book to write is the one of personal accounts, for they are real to the writer (myself) and surreal to the reader. And it is here, where my greatest challenge begins as I will attempt to bridge this gap, to unveil the concept of Youthful Immortality as believable and a genuine possibility for the reader as it was for me. To make this undertaking possible I've segmented my story into three manageable parts. Part One will detail my rise and fall and rise again of the Three Treasures. Part Two will outline my own unique interpretation of the Three Treasures. Part Three will highlight some of my insights and experience throughout the years which will aid the practitioner in their own goals of achieving Youthful Immortality.

Part One

To begin with, my story isn't just about me or about Taoism or even about the Three Treasures, but nevertheless it wouldn't be possible without all three because they are all connected. I believe the seeds of immortality were sowed within me before my birth while the philosophy of Taoism nurtured its growth. My primordial life cycle was completed with the mastering of the Three Treasures which ushered the new beginning of my rebirth as a Youthful Immortal.

As a child, my mind was always filled images of living an endless existence. The heroes I admired as a young boy were the ones who could not be harm and who could never die. My original awe with nature would ignite the flame that would light the way to seek Taoism as a spiritual guide and the Three Treasures as my path to achieving my childhood dream.

Not satisfied in mastering the Three Treasures in my early twenties I went forth to travel the world in search for a 'True Master' of Qi to guide me to my big reward of immortality. I trained under several Qi Gong and Tai Chi masters. I also attended many Qi Gong/Tai Chi conventions and went so far as the other side of the world to seek worthy teachers of different esoteric arts. As I continued my search I remained faithful in practicing my own version of the Three Treasures. In my investigation to find the right teacher I have met several so-called masters and many more who believe they have some special power or other. In the end, my pursuit to find the 'True Master' was doomed from the start. For many years I could not see the forest through the trees. It was not until I finally gave up looking that I could now see my own revelation revealing itself. I suddenly began to notice the vast difference in appearance between myself and the people around me. Since mastering the Three Treasures I did receive my big reward of remaining young; it wasn't until now that I finally realized it.

Part Two

Ancient Taoist scriptures describe the Three Treasures as Ching (the body), Qi (the breath) and Shen (the spirit). Unfortunately, the writings were very vague and were not specific on the techniques and methods used by the ancient sages. The reason is that every Taoist sage practiced their own methods of preserving the Three Treasures. In addition, the practice of the Three Treasures had been going on hundreds of years before the first writings of it. Just like the ancient Taoist sages before me, I have developed my own techniques and methods to preserve the Three Treasures. In addition, I have created my own Qi Gong forms to 1) stir up the surrounding Qi (Awakening the Qi), 2) created my own brand of Qi facial (Qi Gong Botox) and to 3) spread Qi to the entire body (my own Qi Gong style).

Without waiting twenty plus years like I had to check ones progress of the Three Treasures, I've developed a hypothetical 3T's charts outlining the progress based on three models 1) a self-analysis, the 2) progress chart for a middle-aged person and 3) one for a senior/old person. With these three separate models one can visualize their own progress of the Three Treasures in the future.

Part Three

Achieving Youthful Immortality isn't only about restoring and developing the Three Treasures. I've spent a life time preserving the 3T's but I've also spent as much time putting its philosophy and ideologies into practice in my daily life. You see, a practitioner just doesn't study Taoism; he/she has to actually live and experience it to fully understand it. In the end, the practitioner of Youthful Immortality is one with nature and has developed a deep understanding of where he/she fits in with the world. There are several topics and issues that I will narrate some of my insights to the reader which I believe would be a great asset to them in their path to achieving Youthful Immortality. In the end, like any good book I will review everything outlined and hopefully put any missing pieces of the puzzle in its proper place for the reader.

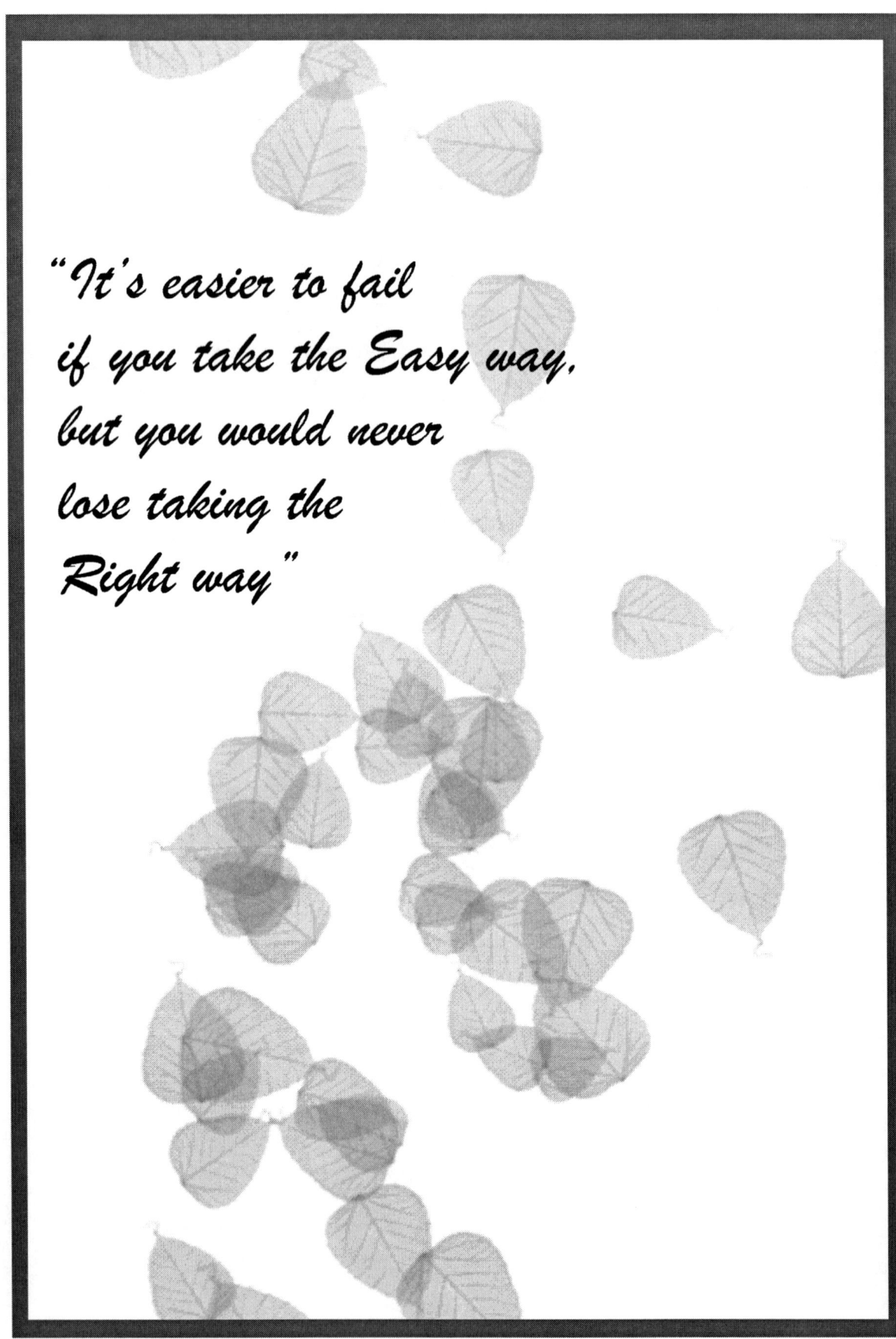

"It's easier to fail
if you take the Easy way,
but you would never
lose taking the
Right way"

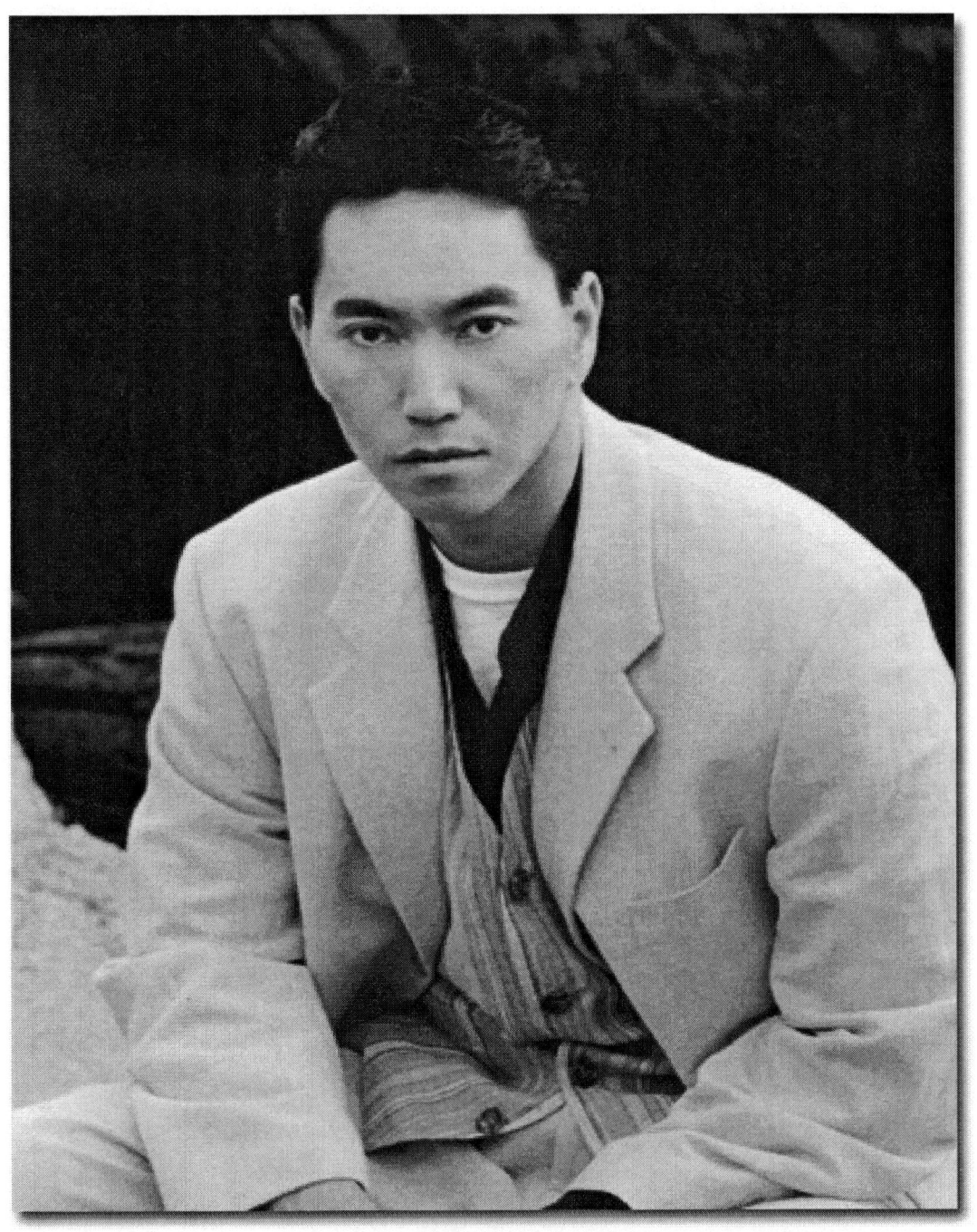

Norm Than at age 21

In the Beginning

"A journey of a thousand miles begins…. By knowing where to go" N.T

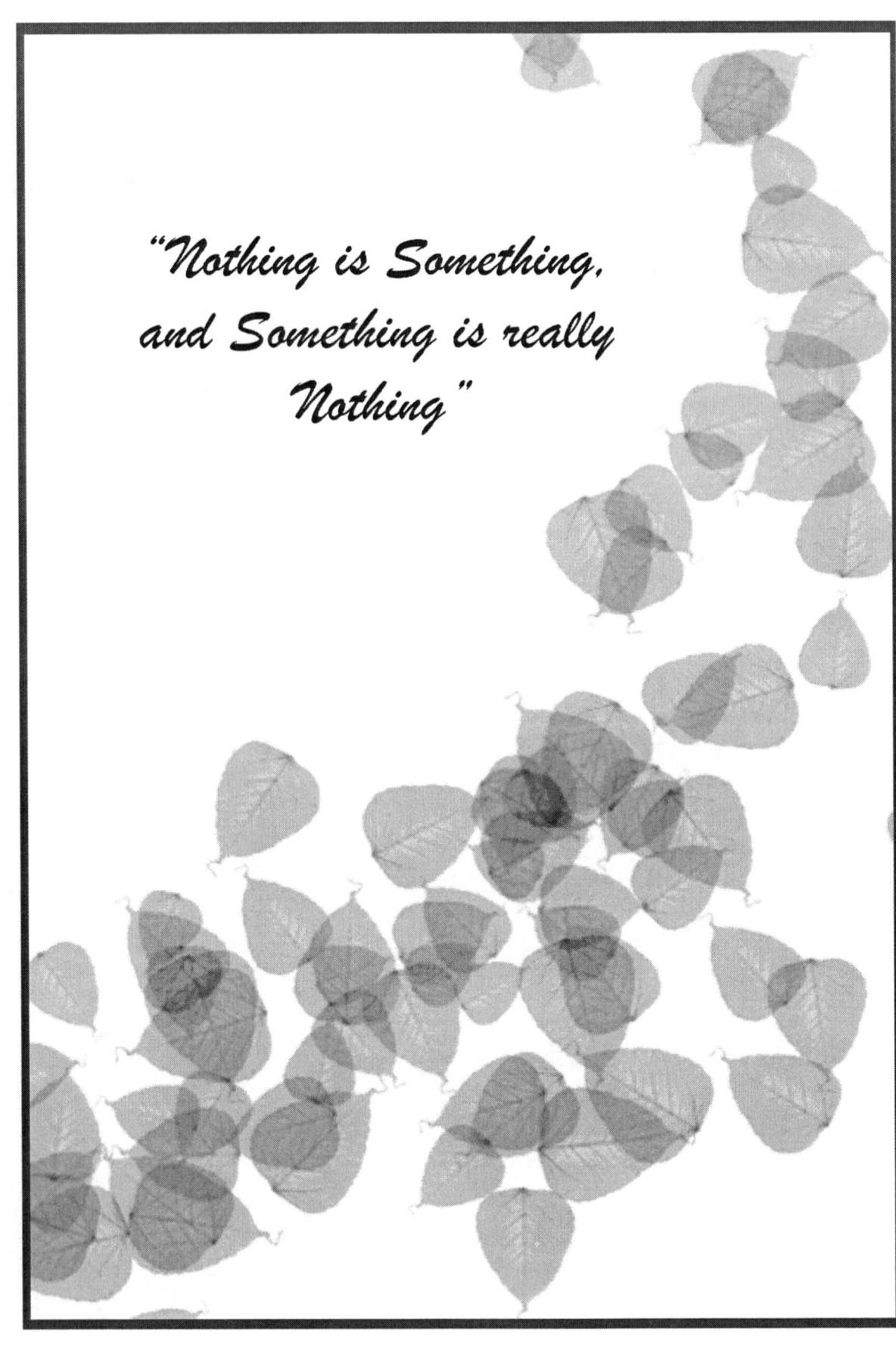

"Nothing is Something,
and Something is really
Nothing"

How old did you say you were?

That question is often repeated by someone having heard my age for first the time. Many thought they may have misheard me or just wanted to repeat the question to be sure. The next reaction is astonishment then a moment of silence to reflect and then disbelief. "No you're not; you're kidding me. There's no way you could be that old. My dad's that old and you look half his age, that's impossible!" are the usual responses. Not surprisingly, I am frequently stopped at security check points, airports and nightclubs because they thought I was carrying false documentations. The person in charge would look at me then the birth date on my document, do some quick arithmetic in their head, look at me again and then ask me to how old I am. Once I have responded they would give me the same reaction like so many others. These are the type of retorts I had always received from disbelievers about my age. Even my friends who have known me for years continue to react in amazement when reminded of my true age. My youthful appearance commonly fools my father (who is getting on in years) into mistaking me for his grandson who is twenty-five. As the years travel by and I continue to look the same as I did when I was in my early-twenties, these reactions will occur more frequently with even more bewilderment.

It seems that time travels forward for everyone else but stands still around me. My psychological, physical and biological makeup remained youthful as my chronological age (my actual age) advanced with time. In the beginning I gave the impression of being eight years younger than my true age. But as seasons passed I started to appear ten, then fifteen and now over twenty years younger than what my chronological age says I should look like. It was not unusual for someone to look three to five years younger then they appear. So in the beginning I never gave what was happening to me a second thought. Through a healthy lifestyle and maybe some cosmetic surgery anyone can appear almost five to seven years younger. It wasn't until I came across looking almost half my age that I realized what a phenomenon this was.

In the past I was afraid of what was happening to me and for many years lied about my age so that people would stop reacting the way they did. I just wanted to be normal and blend in with society. But as the gap between my age and appearance grew wider I knew I could not conceal my age any longer nor should there be a reason to. I realized that there was a greater purpose for what was happening to me and that it must be shared with everyone. So when I reached the age of forty-two, I decided that I would no longer conceal the truth about my age and was no longer afraid of the consequences. I should be proud of what has happened to me because I know many could only dream of the same thing. So if there was such a thing as the Fountain of Youth, I have surely drunk from its well many times over but the problem was I didn't realize it till now.

The Quest to uncover the truth

The first time I ever had my age questioned was when I was thirty-two at the time. My girlfriend said I didn't look more than twenty-three. I didn't take much notice of this because I thought she was just giving me a compliment. It was not until other friends and even strangers continued to make the same comment over the years that I began to wonder what was going on. I started to do a lot of self-analyzing and observing more closely what was happening around me, somehow trying to make connections and come up with possible explanations.

Being Objective and Observant

To find answers that were not subjective and ones that I could honestly accept and live with was difficult. I had to be objective and open to all interpretations and possibilities. I had to set aside any egotistical ideas of being special or having a unique gift that was given to me above all others. I believe that only by seeing pass illusions of self-grandeur can I uncover the true answers to explain how I have been able to remained young as others grew old.

I began noticing that my family, friends and people I have worked with looking a bit older with each passing year. At first the difference was small but increased with each coming year. Some started to have a few wrinkles here, some grey hairs over there and even bald spots where none used to exist. These small signs of aging are insignificant by themselves but together spell out how one is aging and going to look like in the future. The results are even more astonishing when I happen to meet old friends that I have not seen since high school. Their reaction of shock and astonishment are typical with each of them remarking how I never aged or changed a bit. They, on the other hand, had grown older and were showing all the signs of a life well lived.

I have also observed how some people have aged way before their time while some aged well. There are many variables which may explain why some individuals looked older and why some look younger. Genetics, social environment, status, religious beliefs, cosmetic surgery are only a handful of possible explanations. But regardless of how one obtained their youthful appearance, all in the end succumb to aging at some point.

A Taoist Clue

I'm sure I am destined to suffer from the same fate like my family and friends because like it or not, everyone grows old. But in my particular situation, fast approaching the age of fifty I still have not suffered the same affects of aging like so many others. "What is happening to me?" and "Why, at some point in my life have I stopped aging, or stopped looking older?" I kept asking myself. "How am I so different?" I am not blessed with youthful features nor am I born with special genes for longevity (members of my family age just like everyone else). I'm not financially better off than others and therefore can afford the latest medical treatments to live longer. I am not physically gifted nor I am I born with any extraordinary athletic talent. I am not better educated nor are there any social influences that may have benefited me in some way like living in an environment that promoted longevity (in certain parts of the world, old age is revered, unlike North America where is it not).

I am, however Chinese and some Asians do look younger then they are. I have also observed that Black Americans or people with very dark pigment generally hide their aging well because of the color of their skin. But even Asians and or people with darker skin can't escape the affect of aging, no one can.

The Big Event

Yup, I'm just your average Joe, living an average life so what am I doing differently than anybody else? Since I was a little boy I knew I was destined to accomplish something extraordinary. Have you ever heard of people dreaming or praying that something special would happen to them someday and when it does they can't see it or for some reason refuse to believe it? The problem is people in general expect some grand clue or spectacular event (like communicating with a talking, fiery bush, perhaps!) to happen to them. They want their fate to appear in big steps not little ones. But they do not realize that when you add up all the baby steps they turn into a giant leap.

Well, like most people, I was hoping and waiting to see this big event that would show me my destiny. I tried everything and waited and waited but nothing happened. It wasn't until I read with great interest an article in a health journal that talked about how your body tends to gravitate towards your thoughts. If a person was always having specific thoughts about something the rest of the body will seek out to accomplish it. This led me to research my past to better understand my present and foresee my future.

Back to the past

Revisiting my childhood gave me the first part of the answer I was looking for. As a kid growing up in Toronto, Canada, my friends all wanted to grow up to be hockey stars, pop singers etc. something doable but not me. I secretly I wished for physical immortality. Funny thing for a kid to wish for, isn't it? But that was my wish, forever staying young. I was constantly thinking of becoming immortal or accomplishing some form of immortality. When my friends and I pretended we were superheroes, most of them chose either Batman or Superman or some other well known superhero. I, on the other hand, wanted to be like Wolverine. Wolverine was a mutant member of the X-Men; he had super mutating healing powers and a titanium skeleton. When Wolverine got hurt he would heal up quickly and be ready to battle again. His mutating healing powers also kept him young and he did not age like everyone else. Even though Wolverine was only a comic book character deep down I knew increasing one's healing ability and staying young for a long time was doable. Unlike being a hockey star or pop singer part of your success didn't depend on talent scouts, agents, your height, age, appearance, ability or being gifted. Immortality was up to the individual to achieve, it didn't have any man-made rules. I don't know why at such a young age I was always drawn to the thought of physical immortality. A child psychologist would say that I was afraid of dying or getting hurt but I believe it had to do with my ever fascination about the world I lived in. I wanted to live long enough to see and experience every wonder that this amazing planet has to offer. It would probably take several lifetimes to see and experience everything in this world so why not make the most out of this one?

Throughout my childhood and up until when I was a young boy I have studied and practiced various forms of exercises, sports and diets in order to obtain optimal health and well-being. I knew that immortality would only be achieved through my own efforts and NOT through some divine intervention. It wasn't until I started practicing different forms of martial arts that I was getting closer to discovering the secrets of immortality. Like all students of martial arts we are taught about Chi or Qi, the body's life force. Qi was used by the martial artist to draw strength and energy. I have witnessed numerous demonstrations by martial artists using Qi to break boards. What these martial artists were doing was demonstrating external Qi. Impressive as these demonstrations were I knew the answer lied in cultivating inner Qi to rejuvenate and heal the body and not in breaking boards. What I didn't know was that throughout my childhood I was already following the philosophy of Taoism and practicing its esoteric arts of moving Qi without even realizing it. Was I a reincarnated Taoist immortal?

Taoism and Qi Gong

As a young adolescent I was instinctively drawn to Taoism and started studying and practicing the internal martial arts associated with it called Qi Gong. The main reason I found Taoism so appealing was that its philosophy it fit very well with my own beliefs about life and nature and the use of Qi.

What I do know about Taoism is that it is an ancient Chinese philosophy that quickly became a religion and has been the main school of thought in China for thousands of years and still is today. Taoism is attributed to two individuals, the first is Laozi and the second is Zhuangzi (or Chuangzi). Little is known about Laozi who is believed to have lived around sixth century B.C. Laozi was considered a mystical hermit and author of the famous Daode Jing (the Daode Jing is a philosophical work that has launched one of the worlds most renowned religion – Taoism). It is believed that Laozi had written the Daode Jing just before heading into the mountains to live out his final days as a hermit. Chinese tradition has Laozi as the teacher to Confucius and the founder of Taoism. Zhuangzi was actually a real person who lived in province of Hunan, China between 370 B.C. and 286 B.C. Zhuangzi was China's most intellectual mind and was believed to be a student of Laozi. Zhuangzi was a great speaker and advocate of Taoist philosophy. Laozi may have been credited for starting Taoism but it was Zhuangzi who carried message to the people and popularized it. The writings and teachings of Taoism and its advocates Laozi and Zhuangzi were very influential in guiding my life and the writing of this book. I will often refer back to the teachings of both Laozi and Zhuangzi to illustrate some points and ideas I want the reader to be aware of.

What fascinated me about Taoism was its overall objective of living within nature and achieving a happy, healthy and long life. In order to obtain the latter part, the Taoist practiced Qi Gong which was the internal martial arts used in achieving that goal. In short, Qi Gong is a series of slow body movements mimicking nature and animals who have, according to Taoist practitioners, achieved long life. Each movement is accompanied with deep controlled breathing. Each breath and movement is with the intention to gather Qi from nature and harvest it within the individual. This inner Qi is then circulated throughout the body and used to strengthen, rejuvenate and heal the individual. A well balanced person has Qi flowing within all parts of his body. It is believed that a blockage or lack of Qi flowing within the channels or meridians (pathways in the body) to certain parts of the body leads to ailment and disease within that area. And it is also believed that one is able to achieve longevity by having their Qi constantly flowing freely within the Micro Cosmic Orbit. The Micro Cosmic Orbit is the circular flow of Qi from the lower stomach (Dantien) where Qi is harvested, pass the rectum up the tail bone then up through the spine. It then goes behind the neck towards the head then back down the front of the face. One completes the Micro Cosmic Orbit by placing the tongue on the roof of the mouth for Qi to travel back downwards to the chest then back to the Dantien again.

Within Taoist philosophy and religion there are many different sects who advocate the practice of Qi Gong, breathing techniques and austerity practices to achieve longevity. Some believed they could even achieve immortality through the Spirit (Shen) while others believed that physical (Ching) immortality was possible. I personally believe that one can achieve a different kind of physical immortality by remaining youthful both physically and spiritually for a very long, long time called Youthful Immortality. I believe one does not have to grow old while achieving longevity, one can also remain young. Qi Gong was not only a way to achieve a healthy life; the ancient sages also believe it kept one youthful into old age. What is the sense of achieving longevity if you're going to be too old physically to enjoy it?

Immortality

The search for immortality is nothing new in human history. Many different religions talk of sages living for hundreds of years. These stories were deem folktales because there were never any proof or solid documentation to authentic their claim. As a kid I was also skeptical until I read the story of Li Ching-Yun who was reported to have lived to be two hundred and fifty-six years of age. Li Ching-Yun was a Taoist hermit who was born in the late 1600s. Stories of his amazing longevity reached very important Chinese officials who wanted to meet with him.

Li Ching-Yun stayed in the home of a very prominent official who took the one and only picture of this remarkable old man in 1927. The picture showed a little white-haired man whose skin was still soft and bouncy. This is a remarkable achievement in longevity yet little has been heard about Li Ching-Yun. Li Ching-Yun practiced his own brand of Qi Gong called the Eight Brocades which, as the story goes, was taught to him by another hermit who was older than him. What Li Ching-Yun was able to do was nothing short of miraculous and has continued to inspire me to this day.

The Forgotten Truth Revealed

I started practicing Qi Gong and incorporating Taoism ideologies fully early in my life. I felt the effects immediately, for example being more into tune with nature, flowing with the Tao and living a less stressful and happier life. With the practice of Qi Gong my skin glowed, my fingernails and hair grew quickly, I was healthier, never became ill and was able to control my Qi energy at will to rejuvenate and heal myself. I knew achieving longevity and staying young also required me to focus on training my body and mind. So I researched, studied and integrated the Taoist practice of the Three Treasures into my goal of achieving Youthful Immortality. The Three Treasures are Taoist practices of developing the Spirit (Shen), the Body (Ching) and the body's life force (Qi).The practice of the Three Treasures has become a way of life for me. On any given day, hour or moment you can find me developing one of the Three Treasures.

The Revelation –part one

As mentioned previously, I like so many others expected a sign or some grand event to happen to make me aware of the miracle that had already taken place within me. I was first given a clue to incorporate the Taoist philosophy and Three Treasures into my life. It never dawned on me that the reason I looked half my age was because of my practice of the Three Treasures. One always overlooks the obvious! The reason it never occurred to me to put one and one together was that when I originally I practiced the Three Treasures, it was with the sole purpose was achieving immortality. But as the years passed, the practice soon became a central part of my life. I believe my personal goal of achieving immortality slowly worked its way from my conscious mind and into my subconscious mind. I no longer thought about immortality but actually lived the life of a Youthful Immortal. For example I would meditate or perform Qi Gong without even consciously thinking of achieving immortality anymore. Meditating and performing Qi Gong has become so innately part of who I am that I forgot its original purpose.

The grand event or sign I was looking for had occurred everyday (in baby steps) for almost twenty-three years after I started searching for it. When I observed the vast different between me and many others the same age I knew this was the grand event or sign I have been seeking. How blind I was not to see this! The Three Treasures really did work! It really did keep me young, healthy and happy into the prime of my life.

The most natural way humans are aware of change is when we compare the difference between A and B. When we are aware of that difference we say a change has occurred. A change for the better or worse will depend on one's own perception. In my case, I was looking for a change within myself and did not realize the huge difference (the grand event or sign) until I started comparing myself with everyone else. The change, or should I say Non-Change, had been occurring in me since my early twenties when I have mastered the Taoist Three Treasures.

The Revelation –part two

Around the young age of twenty-two or twenty-three I believe I have reached the highest level of the Taoist Three Treasures yet I still felt I had a lot more to learn. I wanted to find a grand master, a janitor/karate master, a Yoda, a Laozi in disguise, a 'true master' to show me the final way to immortality. What I was looking for was a fellow Youthful Immortal like myself. Since I have only begun taking the first few steps on a long journey I wanted to meet someone who has already traveled miles on the same road.

As I spent the next twenty or so years searching the world over for the 'true master' I continued to diligently practice my own version the Three Treasures, which in the end would be my savior. In my search I have traveled to many places, as far as East Asia to as close as the United States and in my own backyard, Canada. I went to several countries in East Asia like Singapore and Malaysia but it was in India where I actually met some mystical Hindu holy men who enlighten me about devotion. These holy men were Yogi Masters, called Sadhus. Sadhus come from many different Hindu religious sects and perform their own unique ascetic rituals to honor their Gods. One such austere act a devotee would perform is keeping the right hand raised in the air, next to their head for the rest of his life. As a result, the right hand is drained of blood and shrivels until it becomes as stiff as a piece of wood, in a sense making the practitioner disabled. Because the right hand is believed to be the purest part of the body it is believed that by keeping it away from pollutants of the earth it will remain pure. Other devotees performed similar ascetic acts like spending their entire life on self-made swings to avoid contact with what they believe is a polluted earth. These ascetic acts may seem like unnecessary self torture to non-believers but these devotees have faith that their actions will bring them closer to divination. The Sadhus all had one thing in common and that was the rebellion of worldly goods and desires. Each carried only the bare essentials for life such as a bowl, a single piece of clothing and a walking cane. They live as hermits in isolated areas and are dependent on worshipers for their daily meals. Many of these holy men practiced various forms of yoga and could perform extreme contortions with their bodies. The Sadhus system of charkas (energy centers) were similar to Taoist Qi cavities which I adhered to, but unfortunately that's where the similarities ended. I was unable to find a suitable teacher but nevertheless I was impressed by their devotion to their sacred beliefs which in the end, taught me to be even more devoted to the Three Treasures. With this experience I felt I was closer to finding the answer I was looking for.

This led me to attend Qi Gong conventions in the California area, especially San Francisco where renowned Qi masters from around the world have been known to attend. I have attended several of these conventions in the past and was disappointed every time. These conventions were always the same, with so-called masters demonstrating their external Qi abilities with amateur acts. In addition, every so-called master was too busy minding their egos with gullible students following them around, which created an environment I was not too comfortable being in. In Canada the Qi Gong healers and masters were no different and I was again disappointed. Many of these so-called masters did not preserve the Three Treasures and half of them didn't know what Youthful Immortality was and it showed in their manner and appearance.

The Revelation –part three

In the end, the masters or healers I had the honor of knowing were not the 'true master' I was looking for. I knew the 'true master' would be humble and kind and wouldn't be a show-off. But after over twenty years of searching I did not find one that was worthy. I was so concerned about finding my 'true master' I did not take notice of the world getting older as I stayed the same. I have achieved so much by preserving the Three Treasures but felt I just wasn't ready. I did not have confidence to take the final steps alone. I felt I needed someone to guide me the final way. Just like all the great kung fu and Star Wars movies I've seen as a kid, I also wanted some great mystical master of the arts to teach me the way of the immortals.

It was only when I realized my own failure and had given up the search that I discovered the answer! The 'True Master' was within me! Suddenly I realized that it was only by letting go of my fruitless search that I would finally received my answer. I guess that old saying is true, 'A person who doesn't fail, never learns'. All this time I was too hard on myself! I should have realized that I only achieved what I have till now was because of my own efforts. On that day my eyes were truly opened to see what was in front of me and my own ears could now listen to the truth, I was the 'true master'! Now I was able comprehend why my life unfolded the way it has and what I was meant to do!

Euphoria, that's how I would describe my self revelation. Over twenty years worth of euphoria came rushing through me on the day I uncovered the truth behind my abilities. I had finally begun to realize my childhood dream of immortality. I was excited, it's like watching my lottery ticket numbers come up one at a time until the last number was called. I couldn't explain the feeling of overwhelming joy, satisfaction and relief. This was the third part of my answer! The first part came when I discovered Taoism and Qi Gong; the second part was when I realized how truthfully the Three Treasures worked and the third part was when I discovered I was the 'true master'. My big reward came in three parts and was bigger and better than I expected but to my surprise it wasn't over, it was only just beginning.

The Taoist Three Treasures

As the gap between my age and appearance become wider it may appear to some people that I have uncovered some form of Fountain of Youth. No doubt I believe that the practice of the Taoist Three Treasures played a direct role in keeping me looking young. I firmly believe that I am not special or blessed and that what is happening to me can easily be taught to anyone else with the same results.

In a nutshell, the practice of the Three Treasures involves balancing the spirit, mind and body to achieve longevity. I have researched the Taoist practice of the Three Treasures and have converted much of the ancient practices to suit a modern world. Why didn't I leave the ancient practices as they were? Two reasons, the first is that in Taoism it is believed that a master cannot transfer his knowledge to his student. Understanding and experiencing ones own Tao (pathway or guide) is a personal experience that cannot be taught by an outsider. Knowledge of a master should only be used as guidelines and not as a hard and fast rule. With that point in mind, my translation of the Three Treasures should only be used as a guideline. What worked for me will not necessary work for you! Everyone is different and each reader has to do his own experiment with the Three Treasures. In other words, my guidelines of the 3Ts are based on someone else's guidelines which in turn are based on someone else's and so on. The second reason is that the practice of the Three Treasures is very vague to start with. For example the practice for the second treasure which is the Breath (Qi) only mentions performing Qi Gong methods to cultivate and move Qi but it doesn't specify which ones. The only documented Qi Gong form was found in a burial chamber of a Chinese emperor about a thousand years after many other forms were created. That's because each Taoist sage created their own unique style or adapted other styles. As a result, there were many different forms developed with their own unique history and application. So we will never know for sure which Qi Gong form is the right one to practice but in the end that really doesn't matter. Which ever form you use should be treated only as guidelines and one must develop his/her own distinctive practice for each Treasure as I have done.

I'm just an ordinary guy who just happened to accomplish an extraordinary feat

As I mentioned before I am not a Master or Sensei of any particular martial art style, I don't have a Ph.D., I'm not a medical doctor nor am I a spiritual leader. I'm just an average guy who instinctively followed the ancient Taoist way of life of achieving longevity. I'm just an ordinary guy who just happened to accomplish an extraordinary feat. The reason I have written this book is to show that everyone can be enlightened, healthy, happy and have a long life. You don't have to hold some special position in society or give up all your belongings and change your name to Roshi or become the next Dalai Lama to understand the gift that nature has given all of us. The gift of enlightenment and immortality is available to all and not only to a selected few. This book is specifically written from a layman's (my) point of view. I have written about my experience with the Three Treasures in a plain, simple and easy to read format. I have limited the use of all unnecessary mystical mumble-jumble; perplex terms and their deeper meanings. I, like many others, enjoy and relate to things more when they are put in simple terms and worded in a way that doesn't require a scholarly mind to understand it.

I wanted to write a book with simple instructions to perform the Three Treasures that I know anyone can do and adapt accordingly. Since this is a non-academic prose, I purposely did not go into academic particulars about Taoism and Qi gong, to do so will only lead to confusion. The fact is you don't have to be knowledgeable about Taoism to appreciate its philosophy and guidance. And you don't have to be a Qi Gong expert or perform a particular style of Qi Gong masterfully to gather and circulate Qi energy effectively.

If it isn't broken, don't fix it!

Too often society takes the simplest ideas and turns them into complex mazes in order to understand and control them. For example, the original style of Qi Gong started out as a simple form which quickly developed into numerous complex Qi Gong styles from several masters. Believing that their Qi Gong style was superior, teachers insisted on proper form, technique and breathing. Everything had to be precise or the student would not obtain the insight the master had acquired. But remember, Taoism believes that knowledge of the Tao (guide) or enlightenment or the ability to gather Qi cannot be passed on from master to student. This kind of experience can only be found within the individual.

A short Taoist story is at hand here to sum up what I mean by trying to know too much and being too precise. "A monk was passing by a small village when he sensed incredible Qi energy coming from a little hut. He went in to investigate and saw a peasant sitting improperly in a lotus position and chanting incorrectly. The monk dutifully corrected the peasant and went off. A month later the monk passed the same village but this time did not sense any Qi energy. He went into the hut and saw the same peasant in the correct lotus posture and chanting properly" The lesson behind this story is – "If it isn't broken don't fix it!" One reason I outlined this story is because I am very adamant about allowing one to follow their own way to achieve the same goals. There are so many so-called masters or specialist in different fields who think they know best. You know the ones I'm referring to; they're the ones who sit in the lotus position, wearing the robes and chains with all the theatrics playing the role of an enlighten individual. I had many bad experiences with these so-called masters. At one time I was training under a Qi Gong master who claims to have supernatural Qi abilities. Upon closer investigation all he had was cheap parlor tricks.

At another time I was attending a Qi Gong seminar where they were serving free Chinese tea. There I met a Qi Gong master whose assistant boosted about how well her master looked for his age through his Qi Gong style. He had trained a lifetime to slow down his aging I was told. I was thinking to myself "I'm almost the same age as he is but I looked half my age whereas he only looked a few years younger than he really was". When asked how long I have been practicing my form I said only a few years just to be polite. "Well, you may look as good as my master when you reach his age if you follow his Qi Gong style!" said his assistant who wanted me to sign up for his classes. I said "No thanks, I'm quite happy with my style". "You are too young to practice without a master, you don't have enough experience to know what you're doing" she replied sharply. By now there was a huge crowd gathering around our conversation trying to listen in. Then the question I knew was coming "How old are you?" she asked. As soon I replied there was silence in the room. I quickly left with my Chinese tea in hand.

In the end, you should trust in your own abilities and instead of being guided blindly by someone with lesser power than you.

Two Things to keep in Mind
YI – Intention
A True Purpose

There are two things to always keep in mind while performing the Three Treasures to achieve longevity, even immortality.

The first is "Yi", loosely translated it means intention. Remember –"Where the mind goes the body will follow" "Where there's a Will, there's a Way" These are not old cliques but facts that the ancient Chinese sages have known for eons. Those determine to open their minds and free it from confined thinking will accomplish anything. Your intentions of gathering Qi and circulating it throughout the body's channels or meridians must be true. If your intentions are less than honest, meaning that you are performing the movements and breathing half-heartedly and not truly believing and envisioning the flow of Qi then you are wasting your time. Your intentions must be strong, focused and true, only then would Qi flow freely throughout.

The second is a True Purpose. *"Why?" "Why would I like to be younger than my chronological age?"* my friends would ask me. Besides the obvious reasons the most profound reason is that to me, this world has so much to offer that I need a long life to experience it all. And it is best experienced when I am young and healthy. The spirit world may already have a seat reserved for me but I am not done enjoying the physical world yet. Most people cannot grasp the idea of staying young throughout old age. Everything must go in accordance to a preprogrammed cycle that they are led to believe. People are born; grow up, get old, die and then the cycle repeats itself. The concept of remaining young and not growing old confuses them and disrupts their preconditioned minds.

Another question may be, *"Why would a person who has low esteem or who is poor or who is suffering want to be immortal?" "Why would they want a lifetime of misery?"* First of all, misery is caused by ones own perception of their situation and of themselves. Once they change their perception then world changes too! Even better still if someone can achieve longevity they would have a lifetime to correct or seek aid to their problem. The world is a wonderful place if you choose to see it that way; besides it doesn't do you any good looking it at negatively. "Smile and the world similes back" You must find your own purpose for staying young into old age with reasons only you can understand and live with.

In the past, it was believed that humanity lived longer than we do now. Our society boosts of living longer than our ancestors but mankind's greatest literatures like the Bible and many ancient Chinese writings speaks of individuals living hundreds of years more than we presently do. Ancient Chinese sages like Laozi were written to have lived hundreds of years and even achieved immortality. Mankind through his own undoing has removed himself so far from nature that he has forgotten how to live as nature has intended. Maybe we are all supposed to live a long time like Li Ching-Yun (two hundred and fifty-six years old). His remarkable story and achievement should have been an inspiration for the rest of us but instead had fallen on deaf ears. Instead of being part of nature like his ancestors, modern man has tried to control it. As an alternative to living within nature and taking the long but sure road to achieve longevity, mankind has taken the quicker and easier route. One may ask themselves, 'Do you want to do things the RIGHT way or the EASY way'. Unfortunately, most will take the easy path. Seeking only instant gratification and results, mankind continues to search in vain for the Fountain of Youth or the magic pill that will give him what he already had but forgotten so long ago.

Get ready, get set..

I don't believe I have discovered all the answers of eternal youth with my own version of the Taoist Three Treasures, only time will be the judge of that. In the meantime I will continue to document my ideas, revelations and discoveries about the

Three Treasures. I don't expect the reader to believe or accept a single word of what I am about to purpose in this book. Each individual is encouraged to be critical and skeptical of any information that they hear, see or read about. In the case of this book, I am only outlining my own personal revelations, discoveries and hindsight into how I was about to stay young, both physically and spiritually, while advancing into old age. My own version of physical immortality may not suit everyone but it has plenty to offer for those who want to enjoy life a little bit longer.

So if your "YI" is strong and true and your reasons for remaining young into old age are honest and ones you can live with, then you are ready to dance in the fields of eternal life. And if you are willing to explore the limits to your own immortality, then let me take you on a journey where only ancient sages dare to roam!

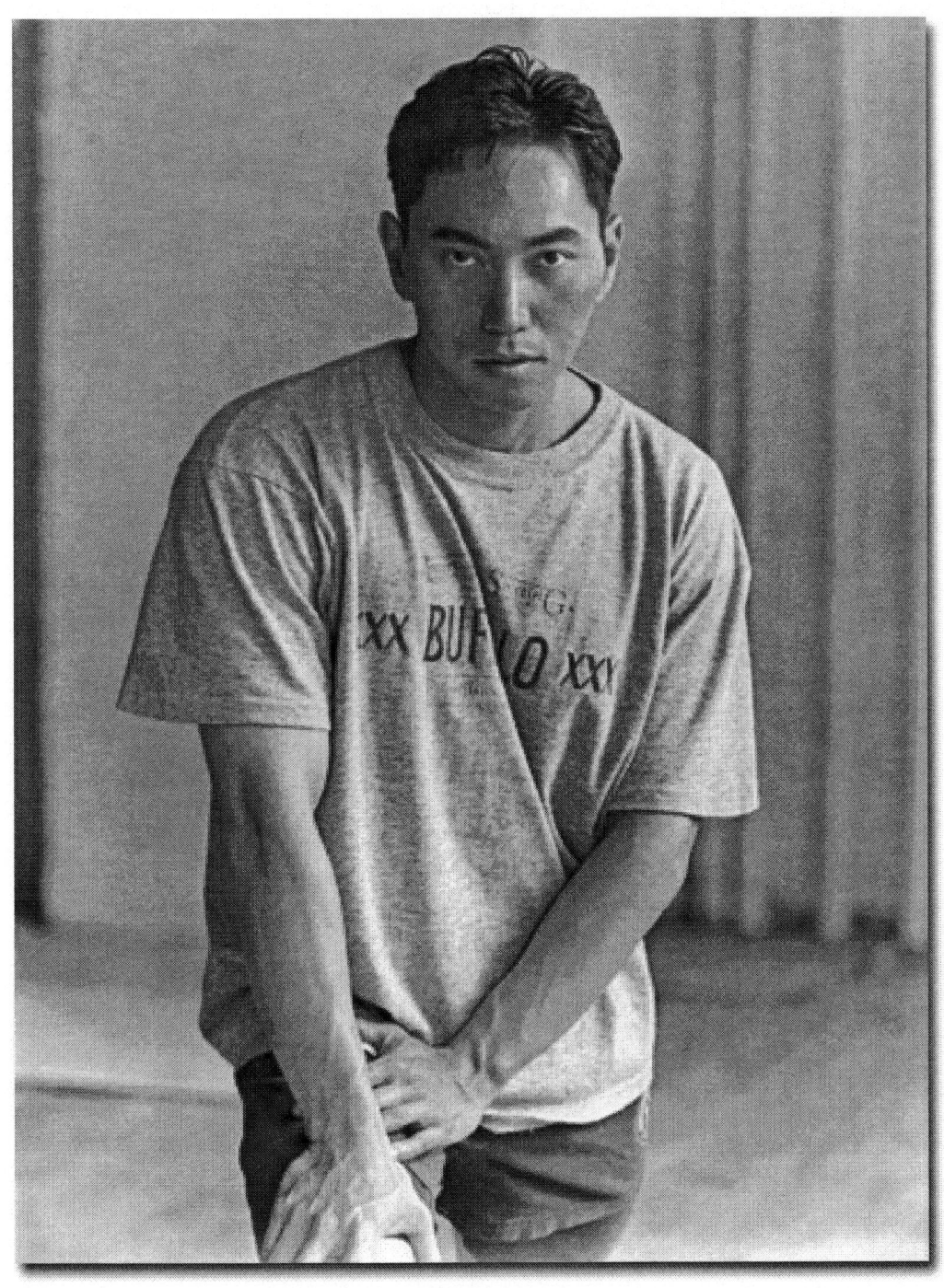

Norm Than at age 28

The Three Treasures

"If I knew back then what I know now, I still wouldn't change a thing" N.T

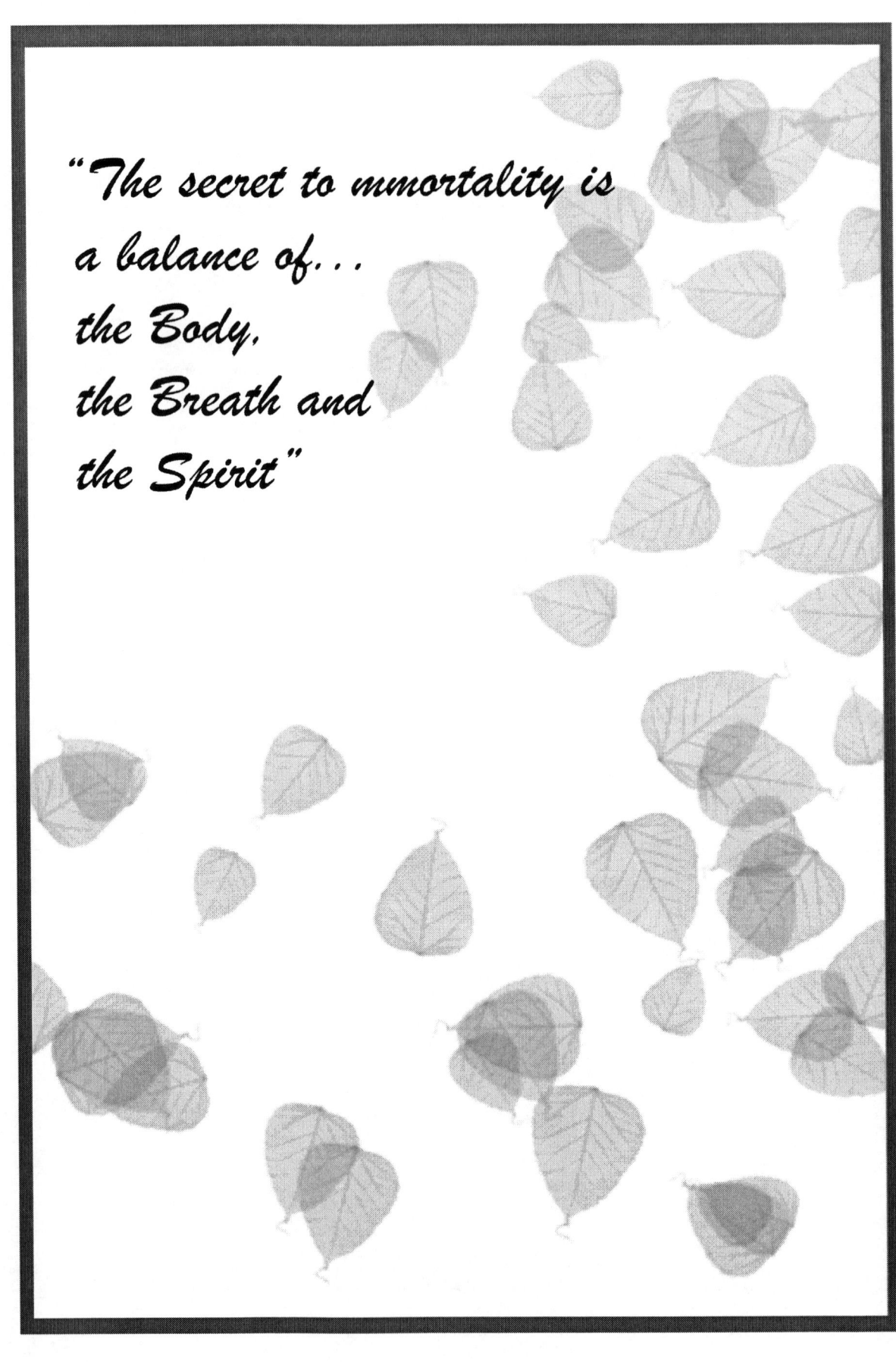

"The secret to mmortality is
a balance of...
the Body,
the Breath and
the Spirit"

The Taoist 3T's

The Taoist Three Treasures

Throughout ancient Chinese history, Taoist followers preached their knowledge of development and restoration of the human body, breath and the spirit. The Taoist called these the Three Treasures; Ching (human body), Qi (breath) and Shen (spirit). They had developed three practices for the Three Treasures and when practiced intelligently and diligently creates a path for health, longevity and even immortality. The first practice was the digestion of herbal medicines and purification of the body (Ching). The second practice was the performance of physical and respiratory exercises to gain breath control and mobilize the Qi (Breath). The third practice is the achievement of mental and physical tranquility through meditation (Shen).

There is no right or wrong way to practice the Three Treasures, everyone must find their own path to performing them. All I can offer is an outline of the three practices I have adapted and developed that worked for me and hopefully for you. Before I begin let me first tell you that these are my personal guidelines and not the original practices of the Taoist Three Treasures. The reason is that the history of the original practices was never written down and what was discovered is very vague and unclear. Researchers are sure the ancient Taoist sages used herbal medicines and practiced physical exercises to strengthen the body. They are also sure that Qi Gong was used to move Qi. And they are quite positive that meditative practices were used to develop the Shen (Spirit) but what they are unsure of is the exact detailed practices and methods of each one. Taoist practice of the Three Treasures has a long history with many continuous changes and development to it. This makes finding the original practices impossible but maybe that's what the original Taoist sages intended. Since a 'Tao that is constant is not a true Tao' then the Three Treasures practices are not meant to be constant but forever changing.

My own version and personal training methods of the Three Treasures that I have developed from the past twenty plus years are guidelines only. I created my own practice and methods based solely on my own persona and experience. I have never been a stickler for following the master/student role, where the student copies exactly everything the master does. I believe that you should learn as much as you can from as many different people who have many years experience and a high degree of knowledge of what you're interested in accomplishing. After that I believe you should follow your own path and be your own master because nobody knows you better than you. This rule is of particular importance because as mentioned previously in Taoism, there is no right or wrong way or a correct or incorrect path to follow. Again, remember a 'Tao that is constant is not a true Tao'.

One will always run into obstacles or opposition when trying to accomplish anything and practicing the Three Treasures is no exception. One obstacle is that it takes a lot of *time* and *commitment.* The second is being *open-minded* and *understanding* of the practice. Time is a luxury a busy person doesn't necessary have when juggling a family life and career. Everyone seems to have an obligation to someone else except for themselves. Everyone finds time to fix a problem (like heart disease) but nobody has time to prevent the problem (eating healthier and exercising). In a modern society where we have many choices to choose from, we don't like to commit to anything in case something better comes along. Why commit years to an exercise program to lose weight and shape your body when liposuction can achieve the same results in an hour. An increase in instant gratification leads to a decrease in long term commitment. We live in a society where we want results fast! Commitment to a rigorous program is passé. The ancient stories of young apprentices training for years with total commitment to their art doesn't fair well in a modern society that is restless and impatient.

We are also a society with fixed ideologies. Rigid and inflexible in our beliefs, it is impossible for us to accept other perspectives on things even when they are better. This results in closed-mindedness and a lack of understanding. Being open to new ideas doesn't necessarily mean we have to accept them but it does lead to an overall better understanding. One can also assist in their understanding by doing their own research. Gathering more than one opinion on anything will always yield a well-rounded answer.

With these obstacles in mind I will now list the practices I have done to preserve the first treasure – Ching (body).

The First Practice:
(Ching) Human body

To the Taoist sages preserving the Ching meant digesting herbal medicines and purification of the body. Since there are many books on Taoist herbal medicines (another name is Traditional Chinese Medicine) and purifications techniques available to the reader I will only summarize my thoughts on the matter. Ancient Taoist herbal medicines are the basis for all Traditional Chinese Medicines (T.C.M.). TCM has evolved over thousands of years. TCM views the body as a whole and sees diseases in terms of disharmony. Treatments try to bring the patient back into balance to restore health. TCM is based on the twin philosophies of Yin and Yang (the dual forces in the universe that is forever changing) and the Five Elements or Phases (Water, Fire, Wood, Metal and Earth). These elements represent the changing seasons and the way humans fit into them. If humans are not in harmony with the movements of nature and if Yin and Yang are not in balance then illness arises. Early herbal formulas were simple and elegant but the later became more complicated. TCM is holistic, meaning that each illness is looked at in its relation to the whole.

I, fortunately, have never been ill since I started the 3Ts so my experience with herbal cures is limited to what my family uses. Since my expertise is in prevention (staying in harmony and in balance) I have used my own mixture of herbs to strengthen key body areas to inhibit the signs of aging.

He Shou Wu

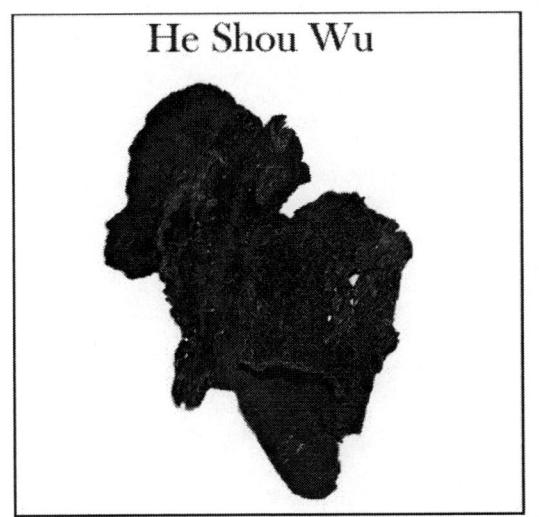

He Shou Wu

He Shou Wu is otherwise known as Fleeceflower Root. This herb is only one of a few herbs (along with Shu Di Huang – Prepared Rehmennia Root) to help the Jing. Jing is known as the Essence of Life. Jing is genetic energy (what you get from your parents) and governs the process of aging. Therefore in theory when one helps their Jing they prevent the signs of aging. He Shou Wu lowers blood cholesterol and protects against hardening of the arteries. It tonifies the liver and kidneys and nourishes the Blood and Jing. I only use He Shou Wu sparingly because overuse can lead to bloating or diarrhea.

Directions - Simply put a teaspoon in a cup filled with hot water, let it sit for half an hour and then sip it. Use only once a day!

Wu Jia Pi

Wu Jia Pi otherwise known as Acanthopanax is especially good for arthritis or the prevention of arthritis. As we age the kidney energy declines, causing weakness in the tendons and bones. Wu Jia Pi strengthens the bones and tendons and reduces the swelling of the legs and stiff knee joints. I have found Wu Jia Pi very useful but use it sparingly because like all herbal medicine complications arise when one misuses a powerful herb.

Directions - Simply put half a teaspoon in a cup filled with hot water, let it sit for half an hour and then sip it. Use once a day!

Male Tonic

Mixture of Damiana, Ashwagandha, Lycii, Amla, Kola, Ginseng (it doesn't matter which type), Cassia Bark, Anise and Oat straw. Mix one teaspoon of this mixture with boiling water. Let it sit for ½ hour and then drink. Take up to four times a day. It is not necessary to know how each ingredient works just that this is a very strong formula overall. This mixture increases blood circulation throughout the body and expands the blood vessels for easier flow. One of the most common male problems is losing interest in sex. There are several reasons for this and one is having too much of a good thing. When a male doesn't give his body enough time to properly recuperate it takes more time for him to get aroused. He can correct this problem simply by getting adequate rest between sexual encounters. The other reason is poor blood circulation within the male genitals. Increasing the blood circulation will certainly assist in curing this problem. In addition, increasing blood flow

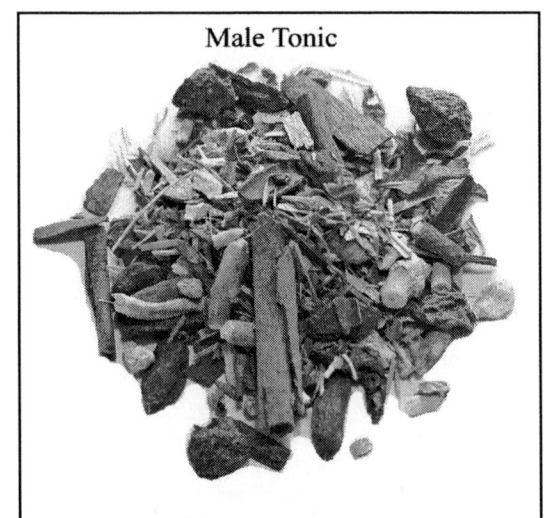

Male Tonic

generates heat within the lower navel area (Dantien) which heightens male arousal.

I purposely chose herbs that I can prepare quickly and easily. Like everyone else I like things simple and taking care of oneself should be simple, right?!

Before trying any herbs please consult a TCM expert. Many of these herbs must be mixed with other herbs and specially prepared, side effects or unwanted symptoms may occur if misused. In order for TCM to be effective, the Three Treasures must also be practiced. Longevity is a combination of many paths that all must be taken.

Purifying the Body

Purifying the body means detoxification of the body of unwanted waste. Taoist purifying methods for the body vary from digesting herbs to fasting to using sanitized cotton cloths to wipe the stomach clean. Herbal remedies have many uses so it is not surprising that the Taoist also used it to cleanse the body. Herbs with high fiber content are digested to assist in bowel movements.

Another method used by the ancient Taoist sages for purifying or removing toxicants from the body was fasting. Various fasting methods are used, ranging anything from digesting only herbal mixtures to going through several days without eating and only drinking water to flush out the digestion system. Another Taoist method is holding one end of a long sanitized cotton gauze and swallowing the other end. As the gauze is swallowed the practitioner would use his internal stomach muscles to contract and move the gauze around the stomach lining. Once finished he would slowly remove the gauze by pulling it back out from the mouth. The Taoist sages also cleansed nasal passageways the same way. Purifying the nasal passage requires one to insert a thin sanitized cotton cloth up through the nasal area down the throat. One would then pull the cloth from the back of the throat. Another method to cleanse the nasal passage ways is sucking up warm purified water through the nasal passages and down and out through the mouth.

These last few cleansing methods may seem a little extreme but the Taoist sages were abet about ridding the body of impurities. The Taoist methods of purifying the body should only be practiced by individuals who are experienced and knowledgeable about Taoist practices. Serious injury and illness may arise without proper preparation and training.

My cleansing methods

As for me, purifying the body consisted of fasting, the taking of herbs and sweating (physical exercise). I only fast in the spring and fall seasons. I use several fasting methods according to the season. In the spring, I switch between a two-day water fast (where I will eat nothing but drink plenty of spring water) and a two-day fruit fast (where I eat nothing but fruits). I perform each of them on a monthly basis on any given week. There is no need to perform the two-day water fast right after the two-day fruit fast. You may alternate or mix up the fast days, it is up to you.

On the two-day-water fast, spring or boiled water that has been cooled down are the only liquids I would intake throughout the day. I would drink about four to seven liters during the day and would cut down on my intake as soon as my urine is clear. When your urine is clear, most of the toxicants from your liver and kidneys are removed. Drinking large amounts of water also cleanses out the natural filters that trap toxic waste in both the liver and kidneys. My two-day-fruit fast would include all sorts of fruits, especially various types of melons which consist mostly of water. Fruits high in fiber like prunes and figs are eaten in abundance to help with bowel movements.

There are many herbal formulas for cleansing the colon but I find taking a mild detox herb on a daily basis is sufficient. The herb I use is called Triphala and is a native herb from India, which I take nightly. Preparation is simple. One ½ teaspoon or less, of Triphala with boiled water into a cup. Let sit ½ hour and then drink. Only a ½ teaspoon is enough to cleanse internal organs as it is very strong (it actually tastes like chalk, Yuk!).

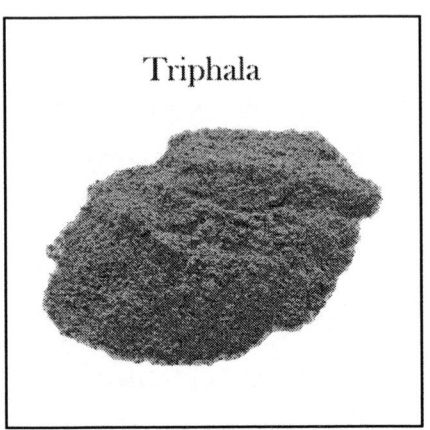

Triphala

In addition to fasting and the use of herbs I also perform high endurance exercises to purify the body, in other words just plain sweating and lots of it! These high endurance exercises include running, swimming, cycling and playing squash for hours at a time. The main objective here is to sweat out the toxic waste through the pores of your skin. You may choose your own aerobics activities but make sure at the end that you have sweated a lot.

The Second Practice: Qi (Breath)
My Own Form of Qi Gong

It's really hard to say what my style of Qi Gong is. It's more like a muss-mash of various Qi Gong forms I have learned throughout my years of practice that have worked for me. My form consists of Awakening the Qi then performing Qi Gong facial exercises and finally my own form of Qi Gong. The majority of movements of my own Qi Gong form were taught to me by Master Wu, from Toronto, Canada, which I altered slightly. When I say my Qi Gong form has worked for me, what I'm actually saying is that I have a personal experience with my body's Qi energy when I do it. The reason I say this is that a lot of books and instructors have given many descriptions of what Qi should be like or how it should be felt. I believe that everyone feels Qi in their own way. Putting a description on how someone should experience Qi only cohorts' people into trying to experience the same thing. It sets a precedence or conventional way of feeling Qi within the body that is not unique to everyone.

The Qi Gong exercises I will outline are what I use to come into contact with my body's Qi energy. How I experience my body's Qi energy will be very different from you and that's how it should be. Though Qi is everywhere and in every living thing we each experience it differently because we are all unique. You may follow the routine outlined in this book, or follow another form or create you own once you have a grasp of the main concepts of Qi manipulation.

Remember and never forget that Qi is your life force. It gives you mobility. Where there is blood there is Qi. Fresh water is clean and pure because it is flowing constantly. Your blood is like water that needs to flow or circulate throughout your body for you to be healthy. Water gets stale and polluted when it is stagnate. In the same sense, you suffer illness or injuries because there is inefficient blood/Qi circulation in the area of discomfort. Qi Gong movements help you circulate Qi throughout the body using your breath, mind and intention (Yi). As you perform the movements you not only bring in Qi with your breath but also using Yi (intention).Yi is probably the most important element in Qi Gong. If ones intention (Yi) is strong enough one can circulate and move Qi within their body.

A person's Yi (intentions) are closely tied to their strong belief and imagination. If someone has a strong belief that he is sending Qi to his right arm to heal it then Qi will automatically flow there. Where the mind goes Qi also follows. This is not at all that surprising that ones thought has amazing power, for thoughts are actually energy waves created by the mind. That is why when you are constantly thinking of something (called your 'dominant thoughts') your body reacts automatically to handle or prepare for the situation you are thinking about. If your objective or aim is to revitalize your entire body and keep yourself from growing old then your intention must be totally focused on that goal.

Using your mind to visualize your goals and to visualize how you see yourself is a powerful tool when performing Qi Gong exercises. As already mentioned, where the mind goes the body follows and visa versa. Seeing is believing and if you can effectively see your Qi energy flowing towards an area on the body that is experiencing some discomfort you will automatically feel the effects of Qi reducing the pain. That is because throughout the body are meridians or channels that travel back to the brain; which enables your mind to quickly send Qi whenever and wherever it is needed.

Awakening the Qi

Before any physical workout you must always warm up and performing Qi Gong exercises is no different. Though Qi Gong movements are not strenuous a proper warm up to awaken the Qi energy is in order. The ancient Taoist sages had many exercises to stir up the Qi within the body. Taoist sages have observed the movements of nature and incorporated these movements in their Qi Gong exercises and warm ups. The ancient Taoist sages copied movements of animals and of nature as they start their day. Each movement has a descriptive name associated with it. For example a Qi Gong exercise called "Bird stretches it wings" was a result of Taoist sages observing birds beginning the day by stretching their wings and shaking their heads; and so their movements were incorporated in a routine to awaken the Qi.

I advise readers to perform at least two or more of the Awakening the Qi exercises I have outlined before starting any Qi Gong form, because by doing so it will increase the amount of Qi you can cultivate.

Morning and Late Night Practices

Between 6:00 am and 11:00 am and between 7:00 pm and 11:00 pm are the best times to perform Qi Gong exercises. It is believed that external Qi energy is highest during these times. Be cautious of performing Qi Gong exercises too late at night. This is because your Qi energy will be heightened at the end of the exercises and if you were planning on sleeping afterwards you will not be able to. Instead you may be restless as you lie on your bed trying to calm the Qi that you have cultivated. Qi is also best cultivated during the spring and fall season because the air is fresher, cooler and filled with Qi. During the winter and summer months Qi is less abundant and stagnant. In the winter the Qi is less abundant because the air is too cold for the body. In the summer, especially on hot and humid days the air is too stagnant and filled with pollutants.

Qi Gong in the Open Air

It's best to practice Qi Gong within nature like in the park or near rivers or forest areas. Stay away from practicing near concrete buildings or in the city. The buildings will interfere or block you from cultivating Qi. According to Feng Shui rules you must be at the centre for maximum energy cultivation. Standing next to a big building only blocks and misdirects energy away from you. Try to avoid practicing in the city as the city pollution will poison the fresh air you are trying to breathe in.

Breathing through the Nose
and with the Stomach

During Qi Gong movements it is important to breath through the nose and with your stomach. Breathing through your nose is recommended because it filters the air you intake. In addition, breathing through your nose allows for deeper breathing and Qi to be channeled to your Dantien (lower navel). Breathing through the mouth creates shallow breathing (breathing through the chest). Taoist sages believe that as infants we are as perfect as we can be and they strive to return to that state of perfection. Infants breathe through the stomach as nature has intended but unfortunately as they mature their breathing becomes shallow and they breathe through the chest. Breathing through the stomach is a way of bringing us closer to nature. According to the ancient sages a calm and well balanced person breathes through with his stomach. On the other hand, shallow breathing represents a person who is anxious, panicky and always in a rush.

Different Qi Gong Forms

Weather you practice my Qi Gong form or follow another form keep in mind that the main goal is to cultivate Qi, so it doesn't matter which form you do. There are many forms that represent nature for example Turtle Qi Gong. The reason a turtle was chosen is that Taoist sages have acknowledged that some turtles have achieved long life and have created a Qi Gong form to accomplish the same thing.

Qi Gong is not only for achieving long life, some forms like Deer Qi Gong, were created to achieve other things for the body like heightening ones sexual drive. So you may use a variety of Qi Gong forms to accomplish many things.

Micro Cosmic Orbit

The Micro Cosmic Orbit is an invisible circuit of Qi within the body with eight Qi cavities located throughout the circuit (see Chart). The Micro Cosmic Orbit, is otherwise known as the Lesser Heavenly Circuit, naturally starts from the Dantien (lower navel) area to the tailbone then up the spine then behind the neck to the head and is completed when the practitioner places his tongue on the roof the mouth; the circuit continues downwards to the chest and back to the Dantien. Keeping the tongue on the roof of the mouth helps keep the Qi flowing as you are practicing Qi cultivation. In

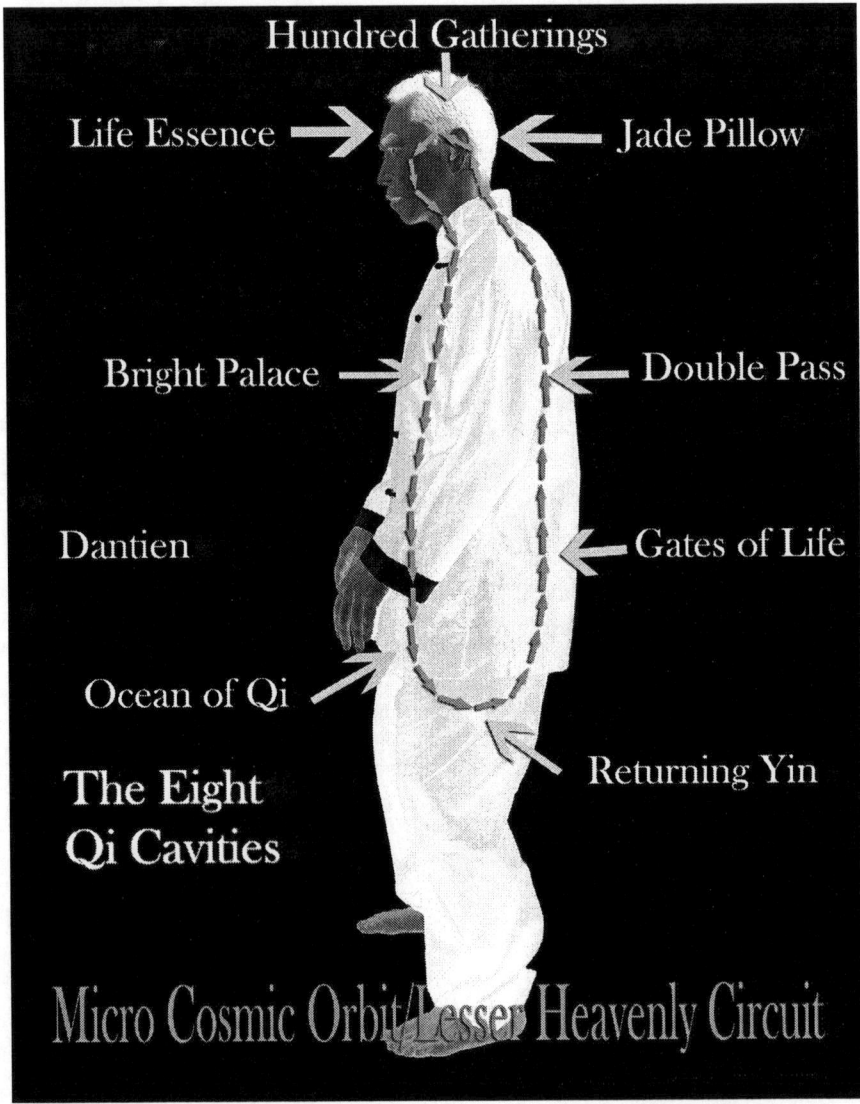

Hundred Gatherings

Life Essence → ← Jade Pillow

Bright Palace → ← Double Pass

Dantien

Gates of Life

Ocean of Qi

Returning Yin

The Eight Qi Cavities

Micro Cosmic Orbit/Lesser Heavenly Circuit

addition, we should try to keep our tongues on the roof of our mouths all the time. This is because we should always be circulating Qi within the Micro Cosmic Orbit (remember, fresh water is always running) and not just during Qi Gong exercises.

Yi – Intention

Yi is a Chinese word that is difficult to translate, the closest meaning in English is Intention but it can also mean belief, imagination, honesty or will and or it could mean all these rolled into one. So if your Yi is not strong and true you will not be able to move or cultivate your Qi. Yi also must be constant throughout your Qi Gong form otherwise you are just going through the motion with nothing happening. The level of Yi is what separates a good practitioner from a bad one. Like completing the Micro Cosmic Orbit (by placing your tongue on top the roof of your mouth), breathing in through the nose and through the stomach, Yi also must be constant throughout your daily activities and not just when you are practicing Qi Gong.

Super Yi (intention)

Last year I saw a BBC program on television about a man who suddenly lost all functional control of his body from the neck down. He had a rare disease that blocked this nervous system from the neck downwards. He spent years in the hospital while doctors tried to figure out how to help him. After a few years of research the doctors concluded that there was nothing medical science could do for him, meaning that he would spend the rest of his days without the function of his body. Undaunted by this tragic news, he refused to live out his days from a hospital bed. His story is one of great courage and great display of Yi (intention) power that I have ever seen. From that day onwards he spent everyday and every moment concentrating and willing his arms and feet to move even though all the nerves leading to those parts of the body were cut off. At first he only focused his Yi on his fingers, just trying to move them. Then one day, all his efforts have been rewarded when he turned to the left side of his pillow and concentrate his Yi on his left fingers and was able to move his pinky finger. That was the start of his amazing recovery. Soon afterwards he was able to move his left hand and then both arms. The toughest part was using his Yi to move his body and legs because they were big body parts but they were no match for his determination and Yi power. After a couple of years he would walk out of the hospital on his own, to the amazement of all the hospital staff.

During the documentary, he was asked how he was able to accomplish such an incredible feat. This person said he had to see the body part he wanted to move and envision all his movements before hand, after that the body just responded! This is especially true when he is walking. He has to keep his eyes on his feet and envision taking each step so he can co-ordinate his walking form. If he ever took his eyes off a body part he was using he would lose all concentration and therefore lose all control. In other words he had to use his eyes to help focus his Yi (intention). His Yi (intention) was like a river that was sent out to reach a certain point. However, that point was block by a huge rock (his main nerves that were damaged). Undaunted and determined his Yi acted like the element water within his body, as it managed to bypass the damaged nerves endings and reconnect itself to minor supportive nerves to give him control. The doctors were astonished because they thought it was impossible. This remarkable feat is a showcase of the power of Yi (intention). Such high level of Yi (intention) must also be present when practicing the Three Treasures in order for success to occur.

Qi Gong summary

As you can see there is a lot more to Qi Gong than just the movements. Qi Gong is an every day and every moment form. Remember YOU are constantly aging, so you must constantly be aware of the Qi Gong principles. The best and easy way to remember and constantly exercise the Qi Gong principles is to incorporate it into your lifestyle. The difference between a good Qi Gong practitioner and a great one is that the great one continues cultivating Qi long after the Qi Gong form is completed.

The Third Practice: Shen (Spirit)

There are many drawings and paintings of Taoist sages meditating alone while surrounded by nature. They are either sitting or standing with their eyes closed or semi closed. This is the ideal conception of the environment and position for proper meditation most people think must occur but this is not true. This is what we believe meditation should be, though it is very picturesque it is not necessary. When one witnesses students practicing Zen meditation (zazen), they all have their legs crossed in the traditional form (sitting with one leg over the other) called the Lotus position. Sitting in the lotus position is not unnecessary! Besides, the Lotus position is a very uncomfortable position for many who are not flexible enough to get into it. And even so it is wise to not remain in the position for long periods as injuries may occur. There has to be something wrong when people strain themselves while meditating! These individuals are only following what they think is the correct position for proper meditation because they see others do it. However, these people sitting in lotus position are no more enlightened then the average guy watching TV all day. Individuals like these are very theatrical and like to dress in the traditional garments, wear the beads, light the scented candles and go the whole nine yards to show off their superior enlightenment and spirituality to others. But in reality, they are more lost then the individuals they are trying to lead.

In truth there is no correct tao (way) to meditation or enlightenment except the one you choose that is BEST for you! If lying on the couch with your eyes closed is your way of meditating who am I to say that you are wrong! I say more power to you for choosing what is right for you and not following the mindless herd.

Other meditation tips!

Many Taoist sages use chants or repeated words like "Sung" in translation it means "Relax". They would say these words out loud and long, like "Suuuuunnnnnggggg" The chanted words are supposed to do just that, relax the body for meditation. The vibrations caused by saying of the words runs throughout the body and calms it. In theory the vibrations are suppose to match those of the body, this equilibrium balances the body. Tibetan monks use similar chanting of words, while meditating, to stay young and to achieve longevity.

Taoist sages like meditating near streams or rivers. This is because they can focus their mind on the sound of the running water. By doing this the mind will not wander. In addition, the fresh running water serves as constant reminder to 1) go to the bathroom before you meditate and 2) be like water.

Now remember a 'Tao that is constant is not a true Tao' so accept these meditative techniques as simple guidelines and not as hard set rules. Meditating is a personal experience so how and where you choose to do it is up to you. I have tried several methods of meditation from various forms like Yoga and the Tibetan Spiritual Chanting but in the end have developed my own technique that worked for me.

Meditative Positions

I use three meditate positions, the Qi Gong stance, the Egyptian and Japanese sitting pose. The Qi Gong stance is like standing limp as though you are a puppet on a string. Your knees are slightly bent but not too much or you would be putting unwanted tension on your thighs and knees. Your back is slightly hunched with the shoulders forward. Your neck is tilted forward bending the neck slightly. The reason for this stance is so that the joints are not locked. This position opens the channels or meridians of the body allowing Qi to flow freely and allows for maximum Qi flow within the Micro Cosmic Orbit.

The Egyptian pose is one where you are sitting down like an Egyptian pharaoh. While sitting down your back and head is slightly bent forward (to open the channels in the Micro Cosmic Orbit). Sitting on the edge of a chair will keep you aware of your position. If you sit too far in you will start feeling too comfortable and start leaning back. This strains your back muscles and in addition, sitting too far back places too much weight on your butt causing it to fall asleep (lack of blood circulation).

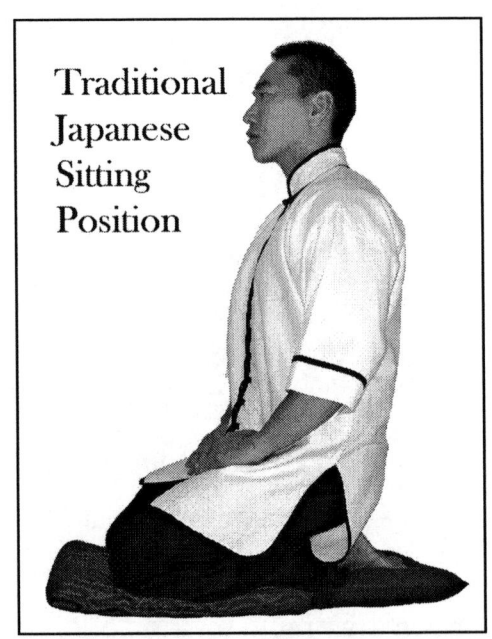

Traditional Japanese Sitting Position

The traditional Japanese sitting position is the most difficult position to maintain for long periods of time. This is because it places a lot of stress on the knees and ankles. However, many Japanese would disagree with me and are very comfortable sitting in the traditional way. If you choose to sit this way, please be sure your knees, shins and ankles are resting on cushions. This will help in easing any discomfort you may feel. Whenever you meditate, first be sure you are comfortable.

Regardless of which position I am in I prefer to place my hands near the Dan Tien (dantien) area as it is most comfortable for me. You may place your hands at your slide but you will find as you meditate your hands will gravitate towards the Dantien. The reason may be is that you tend to move towards your most center point (which is the Dantien).

Trying to hard

There are many different meditation techniques one can follow; ranging from simple to very complex, I prefer simple. Trying too hard to clear ones mind may prove too difficult for most. My meditation technique doesn't put pressure on the individual to suppress images and thoughts that continuously go in and out of ones mind. My techniques actually invites as many images and random thoughts in. I try to analyze each image and see where it takes me but it usually disperses shortly afterwards. I will continue doing this with each thought and image as they come in; and in the end they are reduced to only a few then to one, my most dominant thoughts. As previously mentioned, your dominant thoughts are images or visions you have in your mind most of the time. This is because they have worked their way from your conscious mind deep into your subconscious. Therefore it is most important to make your dominant thoughts ones of cultivating Qi. Remember, where the mind goes the body will follow. If you are centered on your thoughts and images about staying young, an incredible process takes place to the rest of the body; it actually begins to stay young. When we are constantly thinking about something our body's are always listening in and reacting. This listening in includes when you are sleeping, daydreaming or meditating.

Move If You Must

A lot of people are under the impression that while meditating you must be still. Ever witness Zen students meditating? The instructor actually goes around and whacks the person on the back with a stick that he thinks has strayed in his or her meditation. And to add insult to injury the student bows to say thanks and the master bows back to say your welcome. I don't know about you but there has got to be a less painful method to teaching someone how to meditate. If you have an itch on your butt you can't scratch it or you'll break your meditation and worst, get a whack on the back! Nothing could be further from the truth. This type of meditation of remaining perfectly still is just one form of many. And besides, who said you can't scratch you butt? Just because you see others meditating while remaining still doesn't necessary mean you have to also. They probably have parts of their bodies that also needs scratching. It's like the blind leading the blind. Yes, sitting or standing comfortably with the eyes shut or semi-closed and surrounded by nature in a quiet area is ideal for calming the mind and mediating. But if you have to move then... move! What is the point of trying to mediate while you are in discomfort? Your mind will be too focused on that discomfort feeling anyways, so why not deal with it and then go back to meditating. It is not unusual for the body to start developing itches or discomforts while meditating. This is because when the mind is calm it starts paying attention to the body. When the mind no longer seeks external stimuli, it starts seeking internal stimuli. So it is not surprising that your mind starts picking up small internal stimuli like itches but does not when it is focusing on external stimuli.

Let the Inner Rhythm move you!

When you are in deep meditation your mind focuses on internal stimuli coming from your body. Since the mind and body are one this connection is heighten during meditation. Your body and mind become super sensitive to outside and inside energy forces. One particular event that always happens to me is my heartbeat sensitivity is heightened when I'm in deep meditation. I hear and start feeling my heartbeat beating louder and stronger. As my heart beats stronger I actually let the beats vibrate throughout my upper body. At this moment I can feel my upper body sway back and forth with each heartbeat. I remember at first I suppressed this reaction because I was afraid I was getting a heart attack. But I quickly realized that this is the movement of Qi with each heartbeat and I should just go with the flow.

Another time while in deep meditation my hands will automatically reach out to gather Qi that surrounded me and move them into the Dantien area. Although we can't see Qi I believe we can sense it in other ways. Through meditation the mind not only becomes sensitive internally but externally just outside the body. Try meditating under a hot summer's day in the open compared to a cool spring day within nature and your body will instinctively sense the different Qi levels.

So move if you feel like it during meditation, it is just the way your body and mind is letting you know to go with the flow.

Tongue on Roof of Mouth

The Lesser Heavenly Circuit (Micro Cosmic Orbit) within you is constantly flowing with Qi but it needs you to complete the connection in order do so. This means that you should always place your tongue on the roof of your mouth to close the connection and create a natural pathway for the Qi energy to flow. Qi is constantly flowing so you must also constantly flow with it. In addition, placing the tongue on the roof of your mouth during meditation helps calm the mind. Because the mind is constantly looking for external stimuli during meditation and uses all its sensory outlets, like the eyes, nose, ears and tongue to do so. The tongue has many sensitive areas on the top and side of it. These sensitive areas are reduced when the tongue is placed on the roof of the mouth. This also prevents constant swallowing of saliva which also provides the mind with another source of external stimuli to think about during meditation.

Sensory Deprivation Tanks

One of the most unusual devices I have used to assist in my meditation is Sensory Deprivation Tanks (SDT). It is quite a paradox to recommend sensory deprivation tanks to help in meditation. Their original form was called 'Solitary Confinement' and was used to torture prisoners of war. Prisoners were locked in dark rooms with all their senses blocked. They could not hear, taste, see, smell or feel anything within their environment. It was thought that cutting their senses drove the captives mad with insanity.

Today sensory deprivation tanks are like solitary confinement rooms but instead of torturing they are used to relax, calm the mind and help one get in touch with or heighten their senses. These tanks are closed capsules filled with pure sea water about a foot and a half high. Because this is pure sea water any individual will float regardless of how heavy they are. Each is built to only accommodate one person at a time. Each capsule has a door that allows one to go in or out at anytime. In addition, each capsule is light proof, meaning once inside with the door closed all outside light is blocked. There is, however, a small internal light within the capsule for those who wish see. Each capsule is big enough to allow a person to float freely without bumping the sides of the capsule. These capsules are sound proof, meaning once the door is close you will not be able to hear noise from the outside. But there are internal radios that are equipped to play soothing music if one wishes.

The idea behind these sensory deprivation tanks is to cut off all of our external senses and force our sensory system to stop depending on external stimulus and focus on all internal stimuli originating from our bodies. The result is that your senses start to experience your body like never before. For example, you start to hear the sound of your own heartbeat and breathing. Because there is no visual stimulus your eyes starts projecting your thoughts in front of you. Depending on how relaxed you are, you may even experience hallucinations which may seem almost real. Or you may not experience any of these things but feel totally relaxed. Many people fall asleep while in these tanks because it is so relaxing to the body and very calming for the mind. Most people leave these tanks refreshed and well rested. In addition, most experience a heightened sense of touch, sight and hearing. Unfortunately heightened senses return to normal shortly afterwards but sensory deprivation tanks offers a unique internal experience that only deep meditation can offer. After a lifetime of overwhelming daily external stimulus our senses are dulled. Regular SDT sessions can heighten our sensory system back to its primitive state when it was at its best. As we progress as humans we have suppressed our sensing abilities. We no longer needed our keen sense of smell, hearing and sight to trek down our meal. Instead we now only have to wait five minutes for the microwave to cook our TV dinner.

SDT can assist those who wish to meditate as it shortens the time the mind needs to calm down by of cutting all external stimuli. SDT can also heighten our natural senses that are dulled and baldly over stimulated. SDT sessions are quite expensive. However, you can create a cheaper, scaled down Solitary Confinement model that would work just the same. Find a quite, dark, warm and well-ventilated room. Blindfold yourself and place some ear plugs on and wear heavy padded gloves over your hands. The skin is the most sensitive organ we have so to block any sensitivity we may feel wear soft comfortable clothes throughout the body. Now comes the easy part, just lie back and relax.

Practicing Outside in the Dark

Don't be afraid of the dark. Meditating outside during the day surrounded by nature is the Taoist idea of a perfect place to meditate. But another effective method is meditating in solitude in the dark. Yes, that's right! meditating late in the evening in the pitch black of night is just as good. We must embrace the dark as we embrace the light. We should not associate the dark or the night as something evil or less heavenly compared to the light or daytime. Without Yang there would be no Yin. It is believed that Qi energy is greatest between early dawn and 10-11am. It is just as abundant between dusk till midnight. The darkness helps in eliminating any distraction to the eyes. The dark also gives the illusion of being within the Great Void, where nothing is created or destroy but in the midst of either beginning or ending, like the calm before or after the storm. It is here that life and death are the same. It is here that anything is possible. So embrace the dark as you do the light, for they are one of the same.

Progress of the Three Treasures

If one were to try and plot a hypothetical progress of preserving the Three Treasures it would look like the following chart:

1) X-axis would reflect the normal aging effects as one gets older.

2) Y-axis would reflect the amount of time (in this case it is measured in years) one practices preserving the Three Treasures.

3) The **Triangle Shaped-Line** shows the actual age (chronological age) as it steady moves upward with each passing year.

4) The **Diamond Shaped-Line** shows the advanced year(s) one may look like if none of the Three Treasures were preserved (in other words, looking older than they actually are – three to four years to every one chronological year. This tends to occur to people who do not live a healthy lifestyle and usually occurs after early-thirties).

5) The **Square Shaped-Line** reflects the practice of preserving the Three Treasures (the chart presumes that one is practicing the 3T's at a high level).

Detailed explanation of Three Treasures Chart: The sample chart below reflects the lifecycle of a hypothetical individual who began practicing preserving the Three Treasures at the age of thirty. At age thirty-two or thirty-three he quits preserving the 3T's for three to five years but restarted again for the next twenty-seven years.

As you can see the individual on this chart decided to stop his practice of the 3T's around the age of thirty-three. As a result this person started to look older than his chronological age suggests. As his practice of the Three Treasures (**Square Shaped-Line**) declines, the age that he tends to look like starts climbing upwards (**Diamond Shaped-Line**). Now he is looking older than his actual age which progressively climbs up with each passing year. The practice of the Three Treasures aided this person in keeping his youthfulness at age thirty when he started. But three years later for some unknown reason (there are many obstacles in life that will prevent us from preserving the 3T's fully) he has stop preserving the Three Treasures and he started to look his actual age. As the years pass, according to the chart he continues to look older than his actual age. The **Diamond Shaped-Line** (how he looks) has now surpassed the

Triangle Shaped-Line (the chronological age) as the **Square Shaped-Line** (preserving the 3Ts) declines.

But this individual restarts preserving the Three Treasures again at around the age of thirty-seven. As you can see the **Diamond Shaped-Line** (how he looks) also starts to slow down it declines until it meets with the **Square Shaped-Line** (restoring and developing the 3T's). As the chart indicates, the **Square Shaped-Line** and the **Diamond Shaped-Line** meet around the age of forty-seven. This person successfully increased his practice of the 3T's and stopped or slowed down the advanced aging effects on him. In other words, he was successful in putting the brakes on looking older than his real age and is now preserving the Three Treasures at a high level to remain looking like a forty-seven year old. The problem now is that he is actually forty years of age looking like a forty-seven year old. This really isn't a problem if he continues preserving the 3T's, all the lines will meet at his actual age of forty-seven. At this time if he continues the 3T's he will maintain his forty-seven years of age appearance while his actual age progressively goes up. As you can see, if he keeps preserving the 3T's for the next twenty years he will still look and feel like a forty-seven year old but his actual age will be sixty-seven.

I believe this is the Taoist version of longevity and the achievement of Youthful Immortality. However, life is full of obstacles and surprises and preserving of the 3T's may slip from time to time in ones life. With each slip (not practicing the 3T's fully) the person starts looking and feeling older. This may explain why some Qi Gong masters look young and some old. The success rate is different for everyone. Though there are many factors in involved that determines how old one looks at a certain age, the practice of preserving the 3T's will certainly aid in maintaining ones youthful appearance.

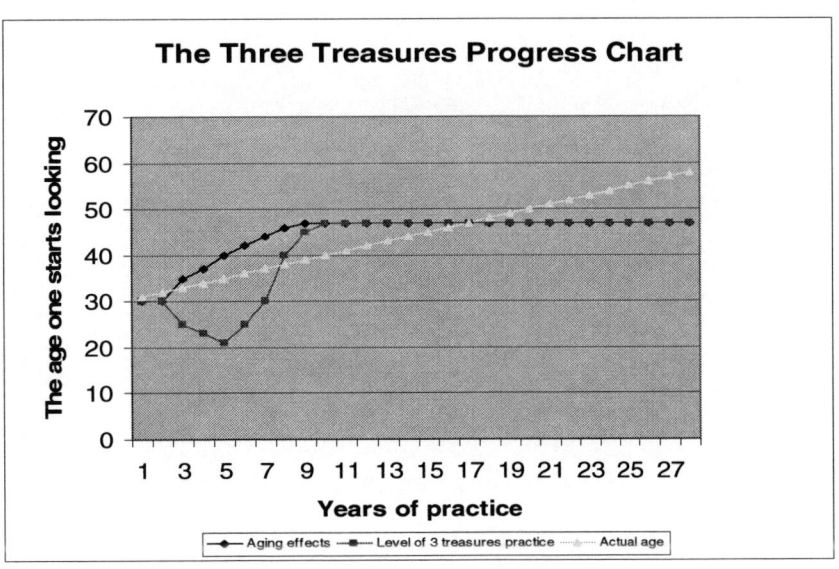

Progress of the Three Treasures – A Self-Analysis

If I were to plot my own progress of the Three Treasures it would look something like the chart below.

The **Triangle Shaped-line** will represent my actual age as it steadily progresses upward like everyone else.

The **Square Shaped-Line** is when I am restoring and developing the Three Treasures at maximum level.

The **Diamond Shaped-Line** represents the natural aging effects. People who lead a normal lifestyle (as opposed to a healthy and active lifestyle) generally look three to four years older than they actually are for every chronological year. This difference increases as one grows older. This usually happens after age thirty or during midlife.

If you take a closer look at my self-analysis chart you can observe that both the **Square Shaped-Line** (Three Treasures practice) and **Diamond Shaped-Line** (aging effects) are mostly in sync with each other. This shows that preserving the Three Treasures rigorously throughout my life starting from about the age of twenty-three has kept me looking like that for most of my life. Furthermore, preserving the 3T's not only preserved my outer appearance but also the inner parts of my body.

As projected on the chart, if I were to continue preserving the Three Treasures at

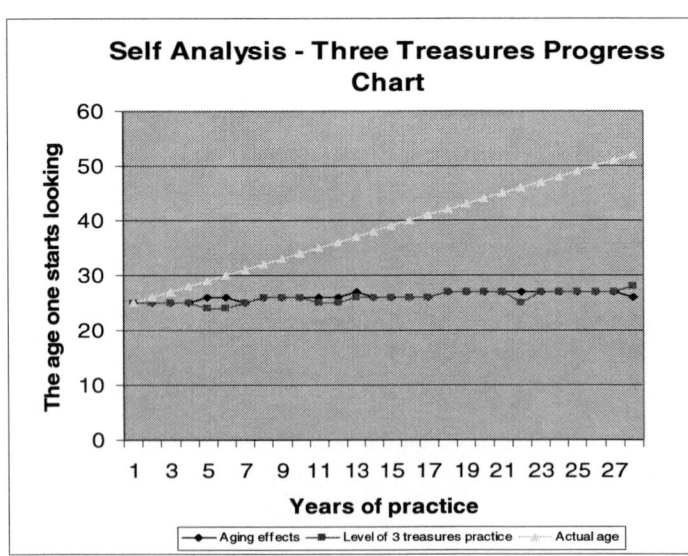

the maximum level I should be able to retain my mid-twenties appearance when I'm over fifty years of age; making me look half my age. I believe I am near the end of the first of two phases of becoming a Youthful Immortal. The second phase of my goal is to look, feel and be physically 'three times younger' than my

actual age and I will obtain that goal when I reach seventy-five years of age.

Progress of the Three Treasures –
Average Joe who has not preserved the 3T's.

When we analyze the progress chart of someone who hasn't preserved the Three Treasures the projected outlook for this person is not good. As the chart below suggests without preserving the 3T's or even having a healthy lifestyle this person will look a lot older than he/she actual is.

The **Triangle Shaped-line** will represent the actual age of Average Joe as it steadily progresses upward.

The **Square Shaped-Line** represents the level of Three Treasures practice that Average Joe does, which in this case is zero.

The **Diamond Shaped-Line** represents the natural aging effects as one grows older. People who lead a normal lifestyle (as opposed to a healthy and active lifestyle) generally look three to five years older than they actually are for each chronological year. This difference is increased as one grows older. For Average Joe he can start

looking older than he is at an early age; it can start as early as in his late-twenties. As the chart illustrates when the **Diamond Shaped-Line** and the **Triangle Shaped-Line** starts separating and getting wider that's bad news for Average Joe. The chart shows Average Joe at first looking only a few years older in his mid-twenties but after mid-thirties these differences are more apparent. When Average Joe

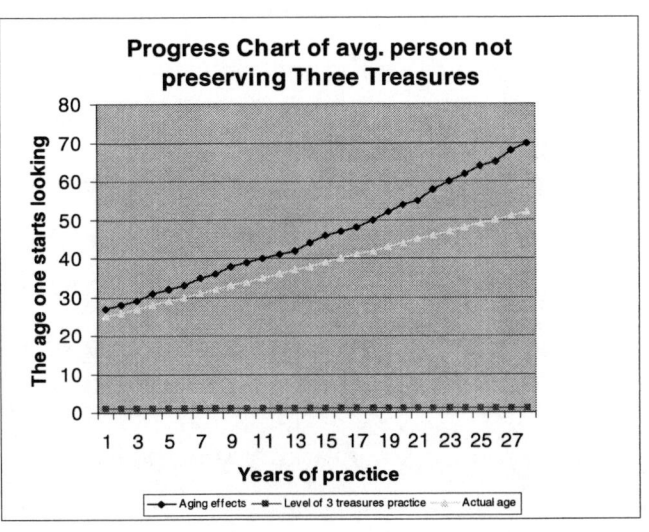

reaches the age of fifty the chart projects he will look like a senior citizen in a retirement home. Individuals like Average Joe represent the majority who opt for plastic surgery rather than practicing the 3T's. Plastic surgery may give these individuals faster and more dramatic effects than the 3T's however, they are limited. Results from practicing the 3T's are less dramatic but safer, steadier and longer lasting. As a matter of fact, the 3T's can work in conjunction with plastic surgeries making the results last longer.

Progress of the Three Treasures – for Seniors

The progress chart for people of old age can be quite dramatic.

The **Triangle Shaped-line** will represent the senior's actual age as it steadily progresses upward like everyone else.

The **Square Shaped-Line** represents restoring and developing the Three Treasures at maximum level.

The **Diamond Shaped-Line** represents the natural aging effects. People who lead a normal lifestyle (as opposed to a healthy and active lifestyle) generally look three to five years older than they actually are. This difference is increased as one grows older and usually begins around mid-thirties.

We will analyze two progress charts of a senior; let's call him Mr. X. Chart One (Figure 1) shows Mr. X who hasn't preserved the Three Treasures at any point in his life. The projected outlook for Mr. X is worst than a middle aged man in the same situation. Even though the middle-man still suffers advance aging like his senior counterpart the difference is less dramatic. This is because advance aging increases more dramatically as one gets older. Not only can you see the difference in their facial features but also on their bodies especially in their statue, bones, liver, lungs and heart. Take a look at the progress of Mr. X in Figure 1. The difference of actual and advance age is almost twenty years for Mr. X. When Mr. X reaches the age of eighty, he looks like he is a hundred years old and the results get worst as Mr. X gets older.

A pessimistic would conclude that is too late to start practicing the Three Treasures for Mr. X and any positive result would be too little too late. Wrong! With the Three Treasures it is never too late to turn back the clock on aging. Remember, once an individual has freed his mind of the confines of time then he/she has eternality to improve, change and grow young again. Preserving the 3Ts is not limited to the young and middle-aged, in fact it is more so for the old and feeble. This is because it is hard to tell if the 3Ts are actually working on a person who is relatively young or middle-aged. The results are not as dramatic and one has to wait till their chronological age advances to the point where they can see a difference. I will use my own scenario for example: If one was to start the 3Ts at age twenty-three and continued to do so until his late forties then reflected back on his progress and saw that he still looked in his early twenties then he would say the 3Ts worked. He would have waited over twenty plus years. Many of us do not have this kind of time and want to see results immediately. But when a senior starts the 3Ts they would see more dramatic results over a longer period of time. Why? Because Qi works from the inside out so their external features would be the last part that is changed. First, the seniors internal organs would be affected then the exterior organs closer to the surface like the skin, eyes, fingernails and hair would improve.

If Mr. X starts practicing the 3Ts at the age of seventy (see Figure 2), at his advanced age he cannot achieve a high level practice immediately but must start slowly. One reason is that the Three Treasures works in a Wei Wu (without doing) fashion. One practice of the Three Treasures involves performing Qi Gong and meditation. Qi Gong is a routine of small, slow movements and meditation is standing or sitting peacefully calming the mind. To someone unfamiliar with the 3T's these exercises appear to do nothing but in fact they are; it's just not apparent yet. Within the Mr. X's body a million things are going on at the same time, Qi is actively moving and re-energizing the body, old cells are replaced by new ones and more importantly Mr. X is rekindling his Inner Nature. Because the practice of the 3T's is so powerful and immediate an elderly must go about it slowly. Another reason is that at his age Mr. X may have settled into a lifestyle and a certain way of thinking and doing things that it may take a while for him to incorporate the 3Ts into his daily routine. So Mr. X must progress slowly at first incorporating the Three Treasures little by little by. When one tries to rush things or force a habit onto a rigid, inflexible pattern two things immediately happen. First, they get frustrated and secondly, they lose patience and quit. But as you can see on chart two if he continues his training he will start to increase his level of practice of the 3Ts and begin to take control of his advance age and hopefully start to bring it down to where his chronological age is.

In time Mr. X will look and feel much younger than his actual age suggests. Chart two shows that by age eighty, Mr. X would have slowed down his advanced age to match his chronological age. Chart two only reflects the average time and improvement an elderly person can achieve; most show remarkable results soon after practicing the

3Ts. As mentioned previously, the effects are more dramatic within the elderly. The reason is that they show more symptoms that we can track improvements from.

Another reason may be that since they have experienced life more than their younger counterparts, their intention (Yi) is more focused and determined, which results in added improvement.

Perception=change

One of the major setbacks with seniors is their opinion of themselves. Deepak Chopra points out that when someone expects to be withdrawn, isolated and useless after a certain age, they create the very conditions that justify their beliefs. Therefore our deepest assumptions of ourselves are the triggers for physical changes. Remember that the body is always listening in on the thoughts of the mind. So when one expects to be old and feeble at a certain age their beliefs goes about to make it so.

As a photographer for a cruise line that catered mostly to seniors I had first hand experience as to how these groups of people viewed themselves. What I discovered was that many seniors had a low esteem of themselves. They believed they were unattractive because they are not young anymore. Old age had taken away their eye-catching looks and replaced it with a worn-out, wrinkled face that they do not recognize. They often shun staff photographers because they do not like how they look and don't want to be reminded of how old they are with pictures of themselves. In fact, many arrive on the ship for what they believe may be their last cruise, a last kick at the bucket one may say, before they leave this world. Unfortunately, these are the same perceptions that are reflected by society (which still doesn't necessarily make it right). Instead these seniors should treat today as the youth of their old age. Meaning that what they do today has consequences in the future. Consequently if they perceive themselves as young, attractive and full to energy today these perceptions gets translated into how they will look tomorrow or ten or twenty years from now. Old age should not be viewed as the end but as the best to come! Therefore it is never too late to turn back the clock, one only has to start with their opinion of themselves.

One thing I also uncovered while being around seniors is that growing old didn't bother them, they just didn't like to look and feel old! Hamida Musulmani, an old woman from Lebanon echoes the same sediments as her senior counterparts. At one hundred and twenty-six years of age she is the oldest person alive. Born in 1877, Hamida still feels well but complains of being old, frail, wrinkled with failing sight. The picture of Hamida reflects her age as she looks old and feeble, with a crumpled, craggy face that had more lines on it than a big city map. Hamida like all seniors can slowly reverse her appearance by changing her perception of herself.

A classic study by Prof. Langer showed how a person viewed themselves effected how they looked physically. The general hypothesis of the study was that if an individual were made to feel as if they were back at a certain time in their lives their psychological and physical being would be altered to reflect their perception. Prof. Langer had arranged to study a group of seniors (between the ages of seventy-five and eighty) in an isolated house for a week. The entire house was decorated in such a way as to reflect a certain time period (twenty years ago). The study group was told to bring only clothes that they wore twenty years ago. Everything else in the house from the kitchen ware to the newspapers in the living room reflected that time period. The study group were instructed to converse only in topics of that time period. In other words, they were instructed to play-act with each other as if they have gone back in time twenty years.

At the end of the study, the study group looked more youthful and their psychological and physical test scores reflected that change. Prof. Langer's study showed how one's assumption about themselves will have a direct affect on how one ages.

Many seniors feel younger than they look and the longer one practices of the Three Treasures their own perceptions about themselves will start to reflect the youthfulness they still feel inside.

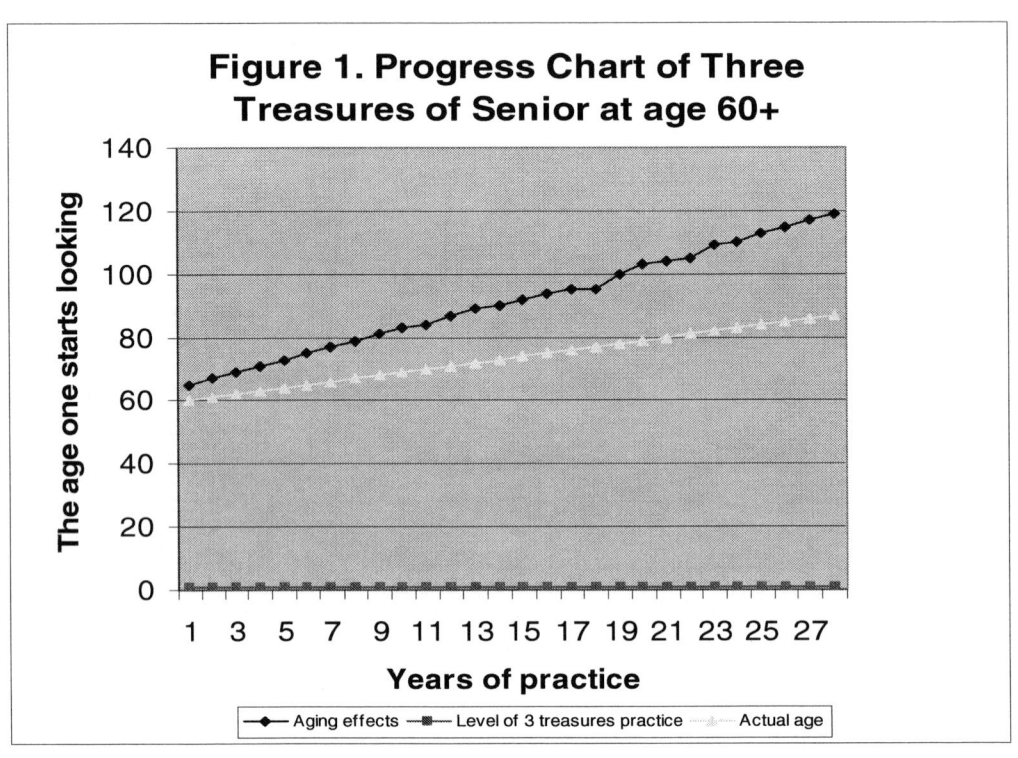

Figure 1. Progress Chart of Three Treasures of Senior at age 60+

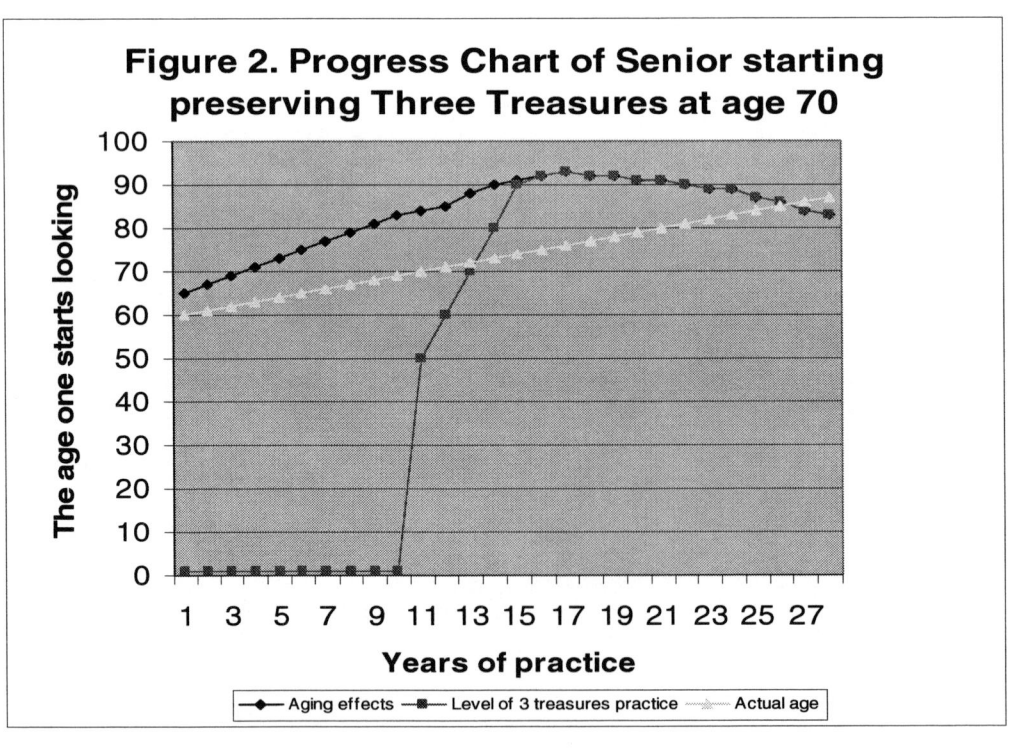

Figure 2. Progress Chart of Senior starting preserving Three Treasures at age 70

3 Ts for Women

Women and water go hand in hand

Were there any female Taoist sages? The answer is Yes! Surprised? Didn't think there were any female immortals in Chinese folktales, did you? Well, there are plenty but they were hardly ever mentioned because most of the ancient writings were created by men. There were as many female Taoist sages as there were males. In fact, women were more successful at preserving the Three Treasures than men. There are several reasons for this phenomenon. First and most important of all, women are more in tune with nature and are more willing to go with the flow of nature. Of the Five Elements (Water, Earth, Fire, Wind, Metal) women are more closely related to the element Water than men! Though all humans are about 90% water it is women who ideally represent water characteristics. Water is submissive and yet always manages to get its way or find its path. When a river is blocked by boulders it doesn't force the rock out of the way but simply goes around it and continues on its merrily path. Guys, think about this analogy for a moment; have you ever known a woman who couldn't get her way? Have you ever gone shopping with your wife or girlfriend and she asked you if she can get something for the house? And you put your foot down and said sternly "No! And to your surprise she sheepishly agrees with you. But at the end of the day you somehow have what she wanted in the back of the car? You now scratch your head wondering "what happened there?" So you see, the Three Treasures are more conducive with the Water element therefore more favorable to women. Even though one needs balance to be successful practicing the Three Treasures it is more helpful for that person to show more Yin qualities such as submission, yielding, weak and water. Though men also possess these same qualities it is women who display them authentically. Men rely too much on Yang qualities such as penetrating, forceful, strong and metal (cutting) and rarely give into their Yin qualities. However, the greatest ancient sages were men which show that some men can have balanced Yin and Yang qualities as well.

Another reason the 3Ts will work better for women is that women have stronger Yi (intention) than men. Yi comes easily to those who are more open-minded and the majority of women are willing to accept or try new concepts outside conventional thinking. Women are more observant, more aware and more in tune with their surrounding. One reason is because for centuries women have been forced into submissive roles. This is, however, actually advantageous because it allows one to watch, learn and understand what is happening around them and gain hindsight to solutions for problems. Men on the other hand are too busy being strong and forceful to recognize their errors. In other words, men do not learn from their mistakes and repeat them whereas women learn and adapt.

Yet another reason is that a female's primitive role was to reproduce. Today that role has changed somewhat but it is still important. And in order to fulfill that role she must attract the male to mate. So it is of great importance for her to look attractive and even better if she can remain attractive for a long time so she can mate more often. Remaining young and attractive for a longer period of time will enable women of today the freedom to postpone having children and concentrate more on their careers longer. Or pursue a career that was unavailable to her when she was raising a family, she can have a second or third career. In other words she can recreate herself several times over because of a prolong life filled with youthfulness.

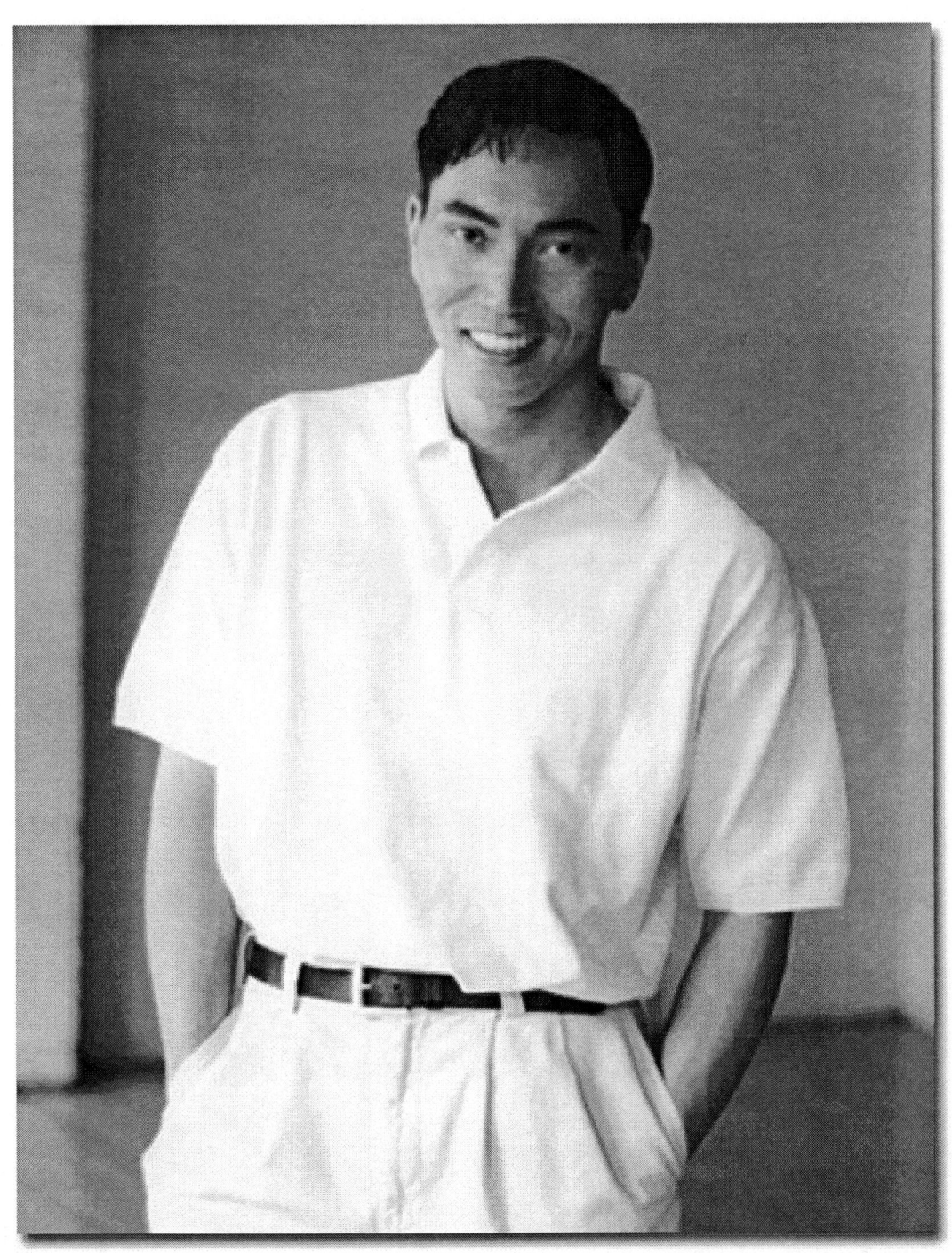

Norm Than at age 32

Qi Gong Routines

"The true reward in any goal is enjoying the journey along the way" N.T

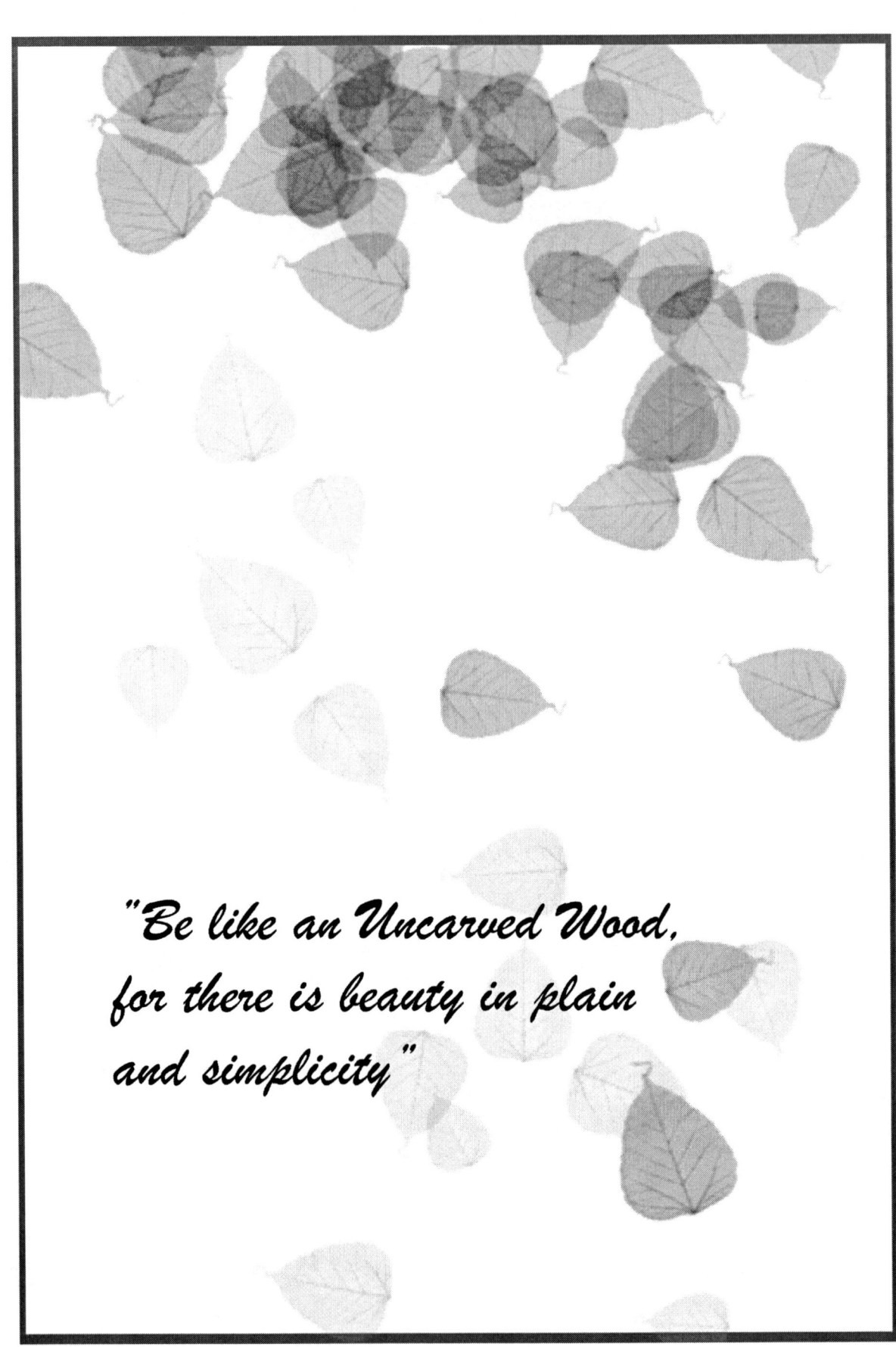

*"Be like an Uncarved Wood,
for there is beauty in plain
and simplicity"*

A Qi Warm Up

A good general rule of thumb when performing any particular exercise is to warm up and Qi Gong is no exception. I have discovered that Qi must be awaken and stirred within and around the practitioner before it can be of any use. Think about filling up your bath tub for a nice bubble bath. What is the first thing you do before entering in? Yes, that's right you stir up the water to mix up the hot and cold water in the tub so that it is evenly tempered. But you also want to stir up more bubbles, the more the better! What is the use of having a bubble bath with only a few suds?

The movements to awaken the Qi are based on ancient Taoist observation of animals in the wild waking up to begin their day. Many movements have been created, some you may have seen before if you ever taken martial arts or yoga. The names given actively describe each movement.

These movements are very good in circulating the Qi within and surrounding you but are more effective when you use Yi (Intention), keeping your tongue on the roof of the mouth and breathing with the stomach. Awakening the Qi movements are not performed in any particular order only that they should be performed before performing Qi Gong.

Bird Spreads Its Wings

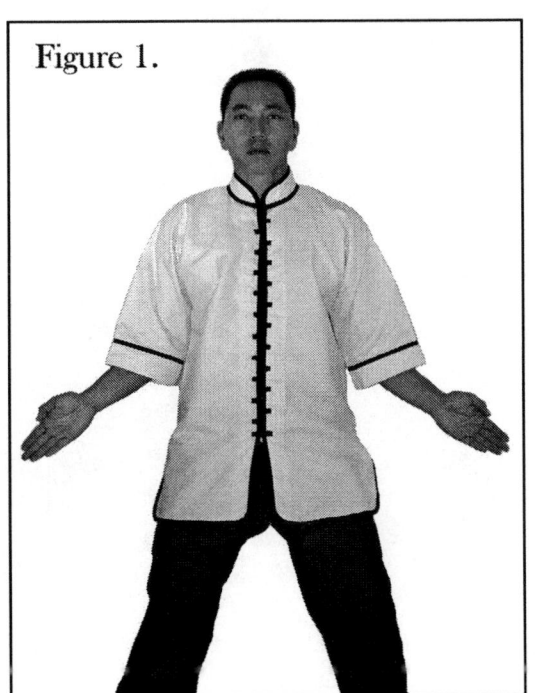

Figure 1.

Stand with legs shoulder width apart and slightly bent with arms to the side. As you lift each arm start straightening your legs (see Figure 1). As you move your arms up spread them out as wide as you can with the palms up. Breathe in slowly as you raise your arms (see Figure 2). Use your Yi to imagine scooping Qi with the palms of both hands. When your arms are at the top of the head, the knees are fully straightened and locked (see Figure 3). At this point you should hold the breath within the Dantien for a moment. As you breathe out slowly lower your arms and bend your knees. Palms are still facing up even as you bring your arms down. Your head should be slightly titled downwards when the arms are down and looking upward when the arms are over the head.

Imagine bringing in Qi from each side with your palms as you raise your arms and pushing away bad Qi when you lower them.

Don't forget to breathe in and out through the nose. You may have your eyes closed or semi-close.

Repetitions: Nine or Ten

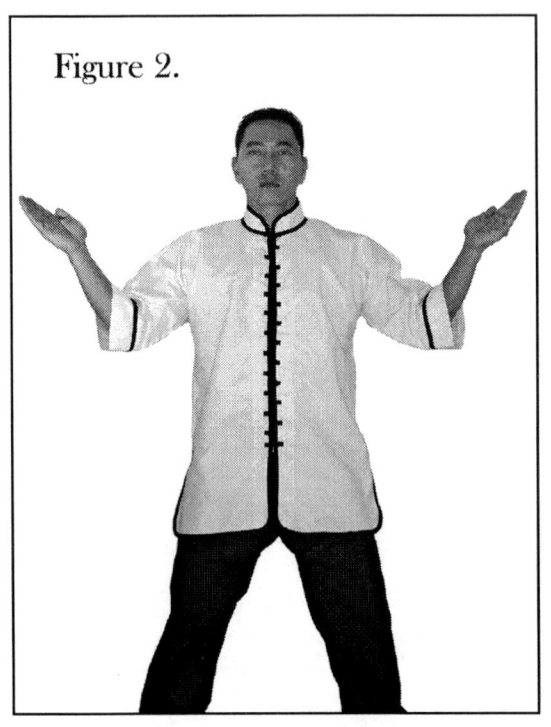

Figure 2.

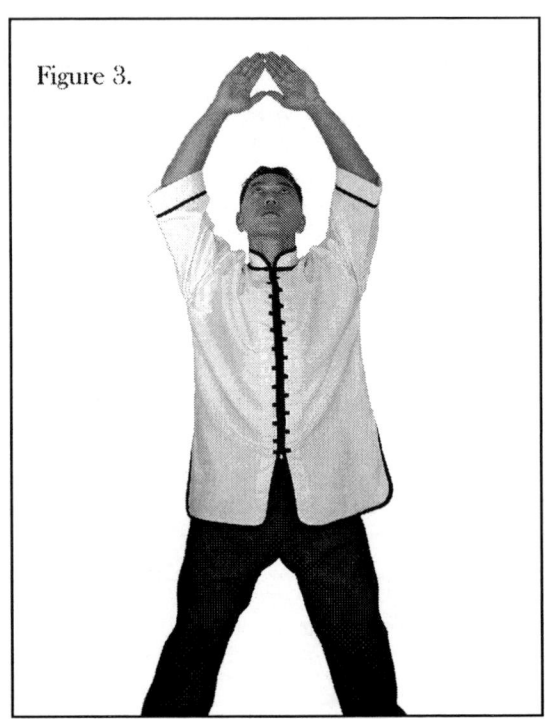

Figure 3.

Horse Whips Its Tail

The movements are identical in the beginning like Bird Spread Its Wing. But instead of bringing the arms over your head you raise them about half way and then make a quick brushing movement in front of the Dantien with one hand and a similar movement on a point at the back called Heavens Gate (or Gates of Life), with the other hand. Heavens Gate is the point within the Micro Cosmic Orbit that is located just

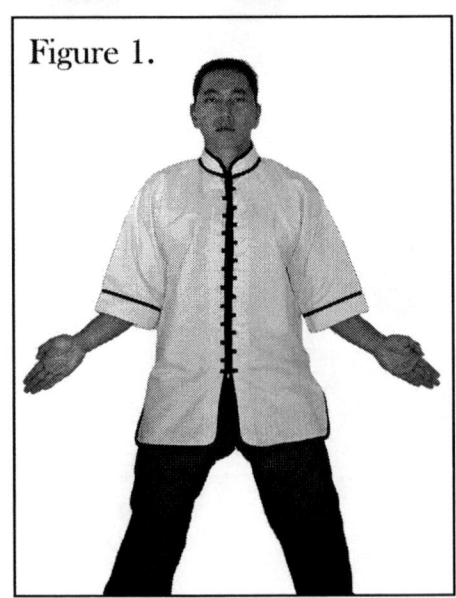

Figure 1.

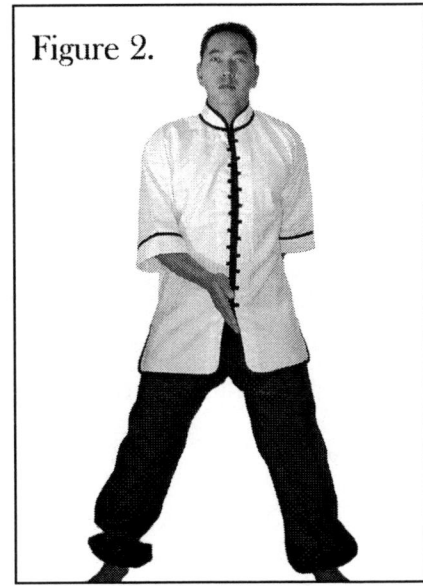
Figure 2.

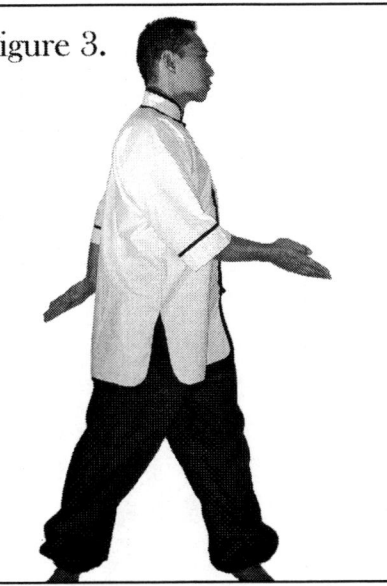
Figure 3.

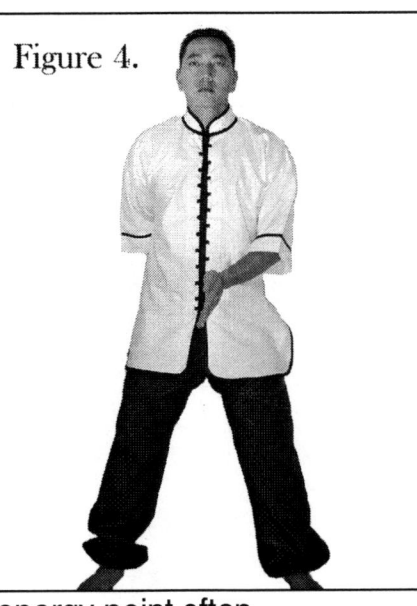
Figure 4.

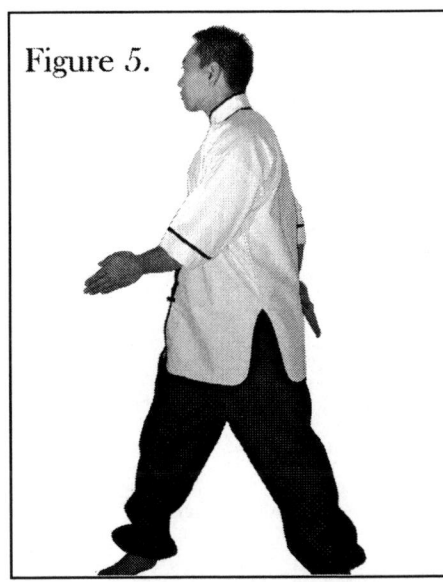
Figure 5.

above the tailbone. It is an energy point often associated with one of the charka energy centers in yoga. Imagine sweeping Qi with your hands in front of the Dantien and Heavens Gate and then switching hands and performing the same brushing movement again (see Figure 1-5). What you are doing is brushing away bad Qi around these areas, in a sense clearing the area for good Qi to enter.

Sweep around the Dantien with the right hand while the left hand is sweeping in front of Heavens Gate. Now swing arms back to the starting position with hands out at both sides. Now you are going to reverse hand positions with the left hand sweep the Dantien while the right hand sweeps in front of Heavens Gate, this is considered one repetition.

Repetitions: Nine or Ten for each side.

Crane Stretches Its Neck

The Crane is a favorite bird of the Chinese because it symbolizes long life. In the morning the Crane first lowers then stretches its neck raising its head high in the air. The Qi Gong form to represent this movement begins with first standing with legs together with both legs and back straight. Slowly bend down and reach for your toes

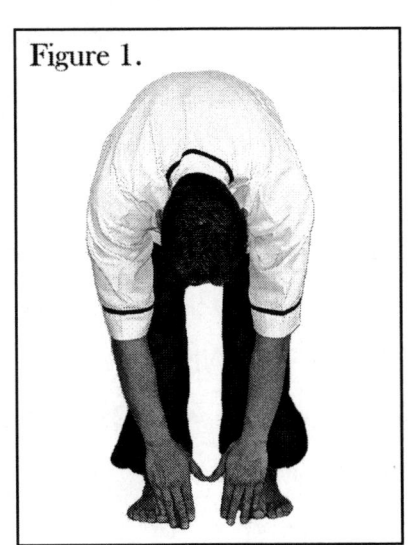
Figure 1.

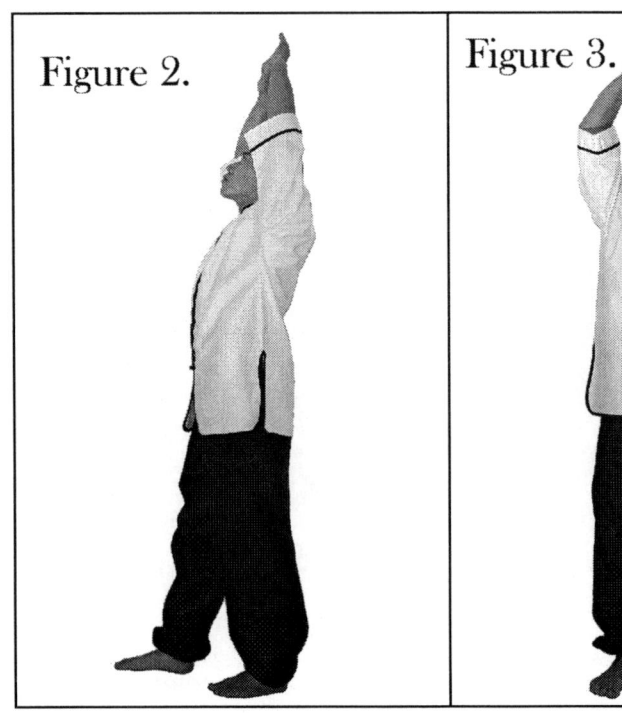

Figure 2.

Figure 3.

while keeping the legs straight(see figure 1). When you have touched your toes or have gone down as far as you can go start rising up slowly keeping your arms straight and hands together in front of you (Figure 1.) As you rise up, take a step forward with either leg. As your arms reach the top, stretch your back and look up in the air (Figure 2 and 3). It is not necessary to stretch back further as this will only cause unwanted pulls or injuries to your back. As you lower your arms keep them straight with hands together. Bend your back forward slowly until you touch your toes, or as low as you can go and repeat the same movement stepping forward with the other leg this time. Remember, to breathe in as you raise your arms up and breathe out as you lower them. Figure 2 and Figure 3 shows the end position your body should be in as you complete this movement. As you lower your body to touch your toes bring the foot you have out in front of you back in line with the other one. Repeat the same movement again but this time switch legs

Repetitions: Nine or Ten

Old Man Washing His Face

This movement is based on how the ancient sages washed themselves by the river to wake up in the morning. While standing, place your hands on your Dantien and breathe in and out. Breathe in again but this time as you breathe out bend

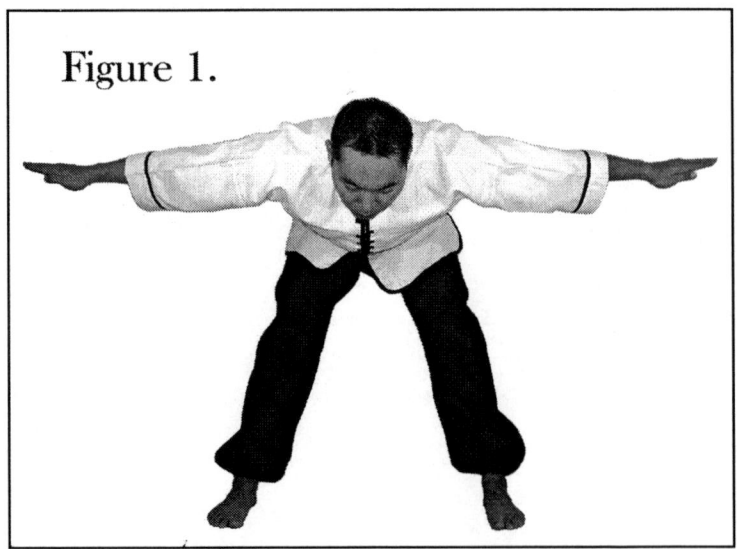

Figure 1.

over keeping your legs straight and stretching your arms to the sides (see Figure 1.). As you breathe out push all the breath out from your lungs as hard as you can while swinging both your arms to the opposite sides of your body (like giving yourself a hug). This movement is supposed to represent an old man splashing himself. (see Figure 2.) Keep swinging your arms until you need to take a deep breath again. When you need to breathe in stop swinging your arms, slowly bend upright and place you hands on your Dantien. Again breathe in and out. On the second or third breath, breathe in and

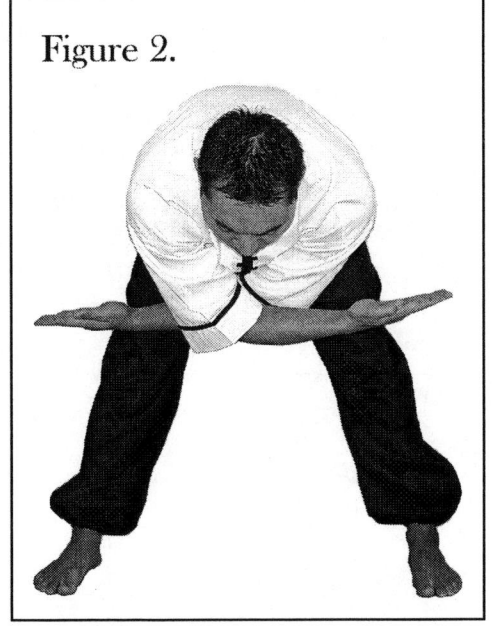

Figure 2.

repeat the same motion. Be careful, this Qi awakening exercise stirs up a lot of Qi and uses a lot of energy. If done too often or if one rises their body up suddenly one may feel dizzy or even pass out.

Repetitions: Five or Six

Sun Rising and Falling

Stand with legs slightly wider than shoulder width. Keep the legs straight. Raise both arms up in the air till hands meet above the head (see Figure 1.). Keeping the hands together start making a big circle beginning with the left side (see Figure 2.). Bend down as far as you can comfortable go towards your left side then down to your left toes (Figure 3.) and then make your way to the middle (Figure 4.) and then to the right toes and up the right side (Figure 5+6). Be sure to breathe in when your arms are at the top and breathe slowly out as you descend towards the toes and in between both feet. Start breathing in again as you make your way to the top. This movement stirs up Qi that surrounds your entire body. Repeat procedure for the right side moving to the left.

Repetitions: five repetitions on each side

Awakening the Qi exercises stirs up the surrounding Qi so that you may cultivate more Qi when you are performing your Qi Gong form. It is best to perform these exercises first thing in morning, because like coffee, they work in getting your Qi flowing internally and externally quickly giving you an energy boost for the rest of the day.

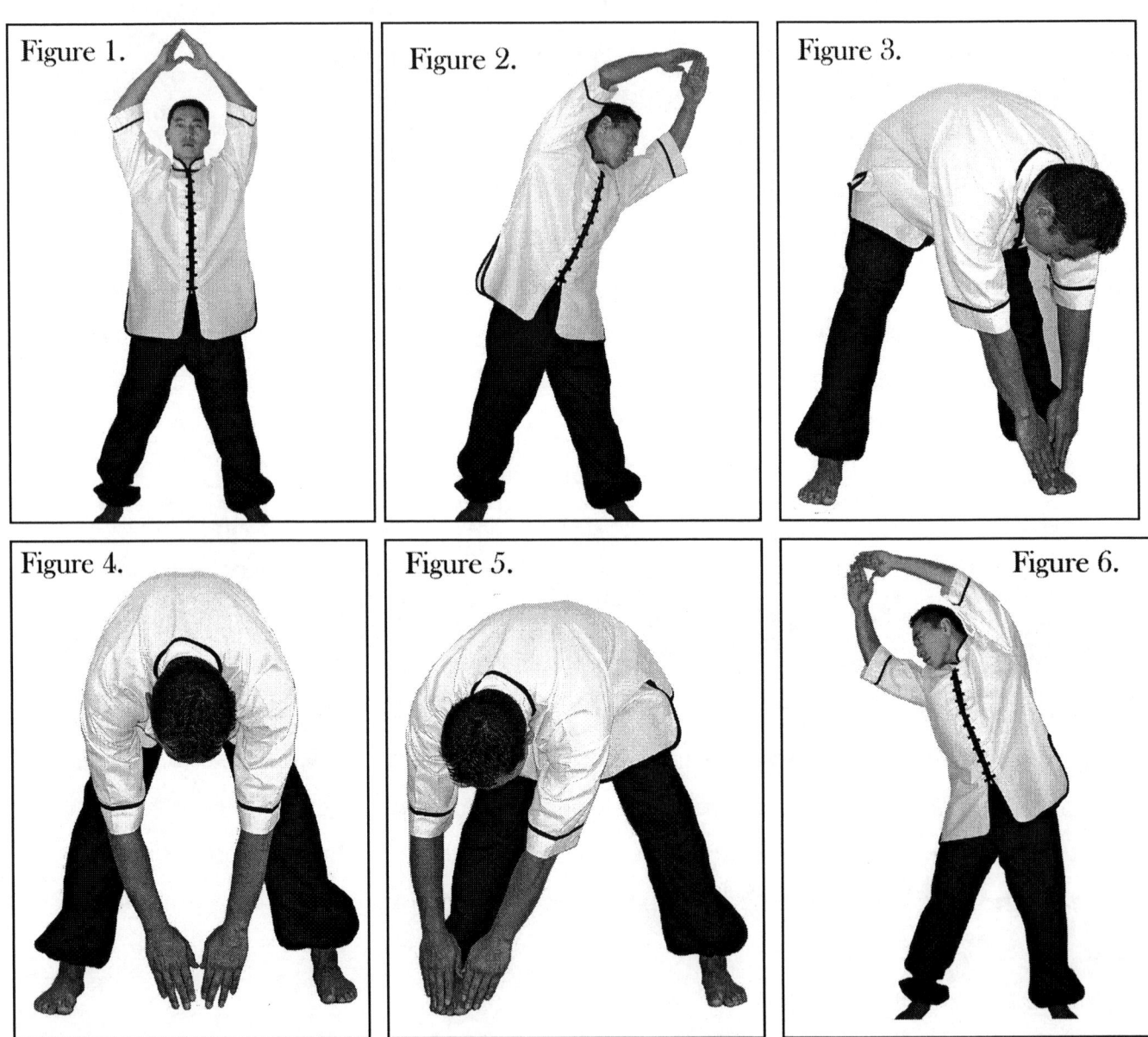

Figure 1.

Figure 2.

Figure 3.

Figure 4.

Figure 5.

Figure 6.

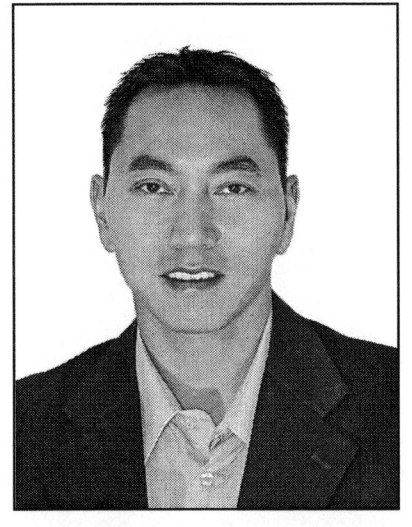

Qi Gong Facial Exercises

Your face is the first area everyone looks at when trying to determine your age. You may have a well tone body with silky smooth skin like a twenty-year old but if your face reflects your true age it doesn't matter how great your body is.

I have developed several Qi Gong exercises you can perform on your face like you do with the muscles on your body. You can actually tone your face like the rest of body to keep it wrinkle free and from sagging. These Qi Gong Facial exercises not only tone and shape your face; it also increases blood circulation in the facial area, giving you a healthy glow. Qi Gong Facial exercises also increases the collagen production around your face making your skin supple and decreasing the chances of developing wrinkles.

There are many facial exercises one can do to tone up the face to prevent and reduce wrinkles but there are only seven essential facial exercises that must be done. I have developed seven Qi Gong facial exercises that concentrate on seven main areas on the face that draw the most attention (see Figure 1). These seven points are located on the middle of the face forming an oval-shaped area. Within this oval-shaped area is where people's eyes tend to be drawn to. It is the main area where people make their first impression of how old you are.

When performing Qi Gong facial exercises there are 5 things to keep in mind.

1-Try to perform facial exercises once in the

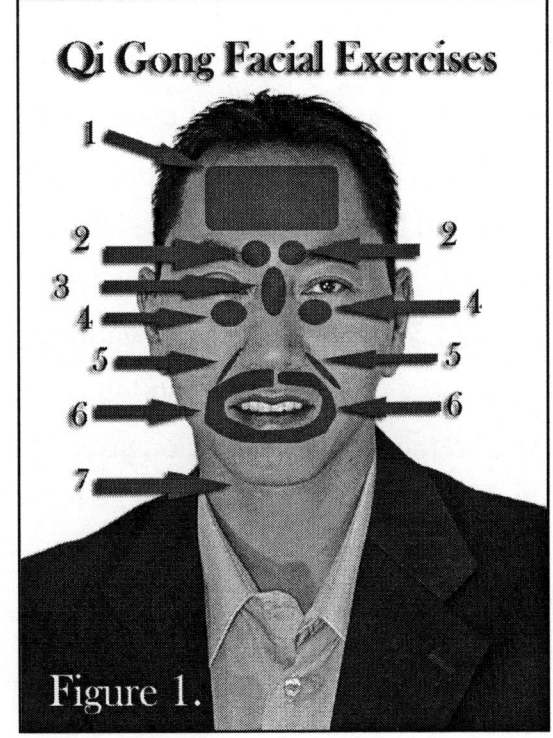

Figure 1.

morning and once before going to bed.

2-Perform at least six to ten repetitions (each repetition for the count of six to ten seconds) for each exercise and four sets each. For example one set will include six to ten repetitions with each repetition for the count of six to ten seconds.

3-For better results try to get a good night sleep.

4-Be careful how you lay your face on the pillow, try not to squish or contort your face. Lines or wrinkles may appear when the face is pressed awkwardly on either a pillow or whatever your head is resting on.

5-Keep your tongue on the roof of the mouth. As difficult and awkward as it may seem, keeping your tongue on the roof of your mouth completes the Lesser Heavenly Circuit, which aids in sending Qi and blood to your facial area. When performing each repetition do not forget that you are still sending Qi to that area so we must always try to complete the Lesser Heavenly Circuit when we can.

Qi Gong Facial Exercise 1. The first facial exercise involves the muscles on the forehead (musculus frontalis). The musculus frontalis or forehead muscles lift the eyebrows and pulls the scalp forward. Constant lifting of the eyebrows creates creases or lines on the forehead which makes the individual older than he/she is.

Exercise: Raise both hands near the forehead. Place the first three fingers of each hand on the forehead, separate them slightly matching them up with the fingers of the other hand. As you attempt to raise your eyebrows, the surface tissue on your forehead will want to fold. Keep your fingers placed throughout your forehead and prevent the forehead facial tissue from rising and folding. Imagine the surface skin on your forehead being a carpet on the floor. When both ends of the carpet are moved in together, the carpet begins to fold over at various points. Imagine your fingers on different areas of the carpet pushing down on the areas that start to fold to keep it flat on the ground. You should feel some tension on your forehead while you are trying to raise your eyebrows. This Qi Gong exercise prevents lines from developing across your forehead. In addition, as you use Yi (intention) to send Qi onto your forehead you are also activating collagen cells to reproduce therefore keeping your skin supple.

After a count of four to six seconds relax the tension and bring your forehead muscles back to its normal position. Keep your fingers in the same position. Breathe in more Qi and repeat the procedure. Perform Four Sets of six to ten repetitions with a count of six to ten seconds for each rep. Don't forget to use Yi to send Qi to the forehead each time.

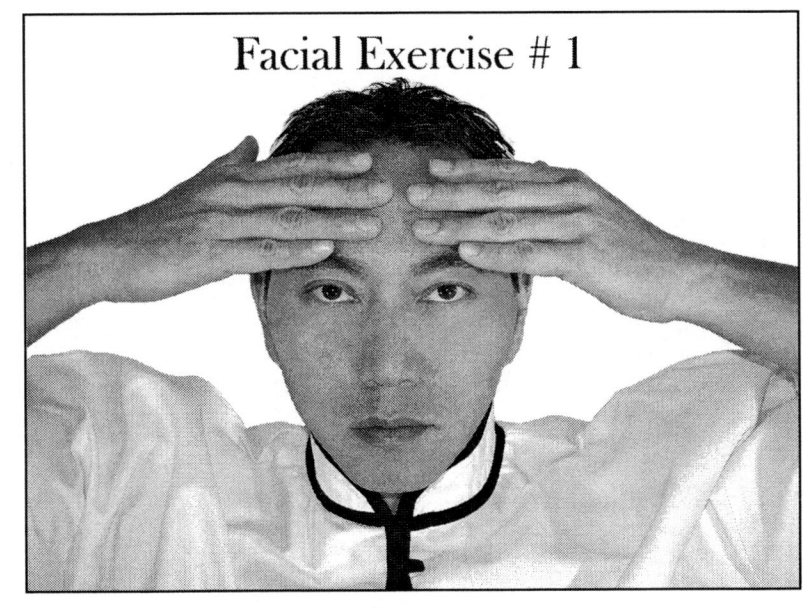

Facial Exercise # 1

Facial Exercise 2. The second facial exercise focuses on the small muscles at the corner of each eyebrow called musculus corrugator glabellae and when pull together they form frown lines. Frown lines are lines between each eyebrow, just over the bridge of the nose. Frown lines are created each time you frown or squint. You may frown when you're mad or when exercising. In either case what happens is that you end up with deep permanent lines between your eyebrows making you seem mad or stressed, or concern all the time even when you're not.

Exercise: Place each index finger at the edge of where the frown line begin to occur. Attempt to frown (bring both eyebrows closer together) but keep your fingers in place to prevent the frown line from occurring. In all of my Qi Gong facial exercises be sure you are using Yi (intention) to send Qi to that area you are working on.

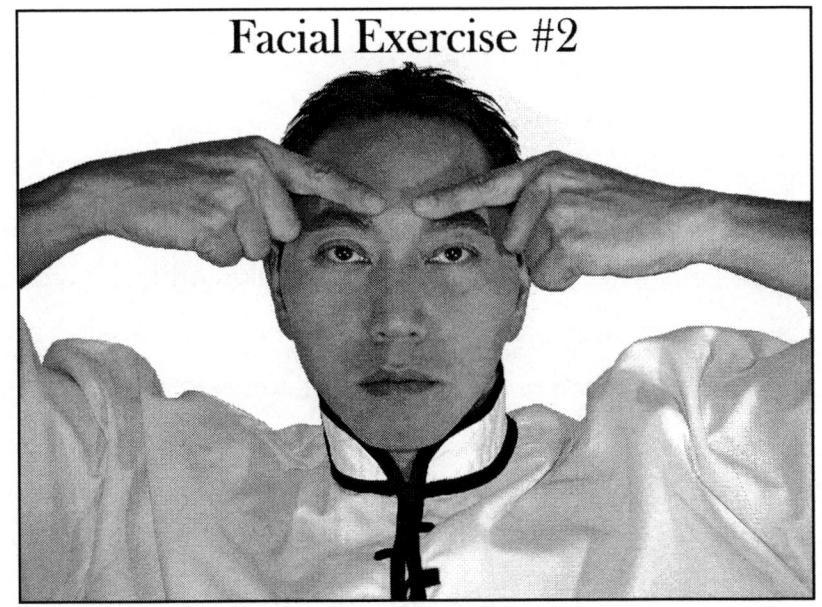

Facial Exercise #2

Hold for six to ten seconds now relax the tension and bring your eyebrows back to its normal position. Keep your fingers in the same position. Breathe in more Qi and repeat the procedure.

Perform Four Sets of six to ten repetitions with a count of six to ten seconds.

Facial Exercise 3. The third facial exercise focuses on the muscles on the bridge of the nose called musculus levator labii superioris. Lines form around this area when you squint your nose. You squint your nose when you smell something bad or when you want to express your dislike of something.

Exercise: Place each index finger from both hands on each side of the bridge of the nose. Keeping the fingers in place try to squint your nose as if you dislike the smell of something. Don't let the lines on the bridge of the nose form. You will feel the tension in the middle of the bridge of the nose. Again use Yi (intention) to send Qi to that area.

Hold for six to ten seconds now relax the tension and let the muscles surrounding the nostrils set

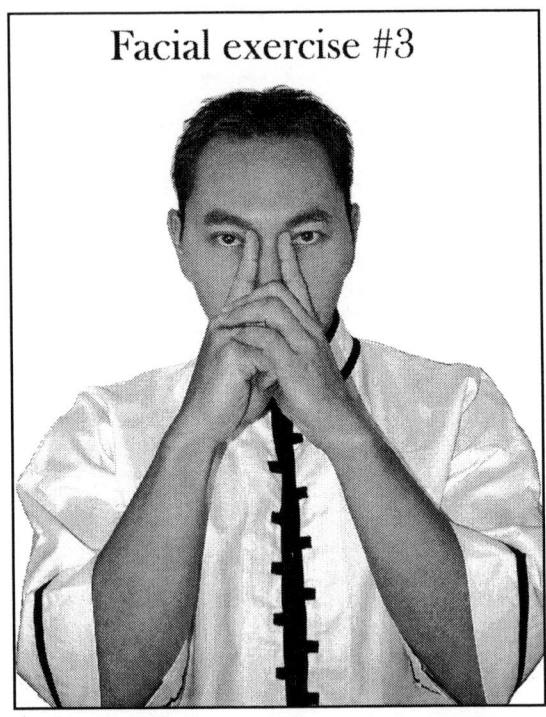

Facial exercise #3

back to its normal position. Keep your fingers in the same position. Breathe in more Qi and repeat the procedure.

Perform Four Sets of six to ten repetitions with a count of six to ten seconds.

Facial Exercise 4. The fourth facial exercise focuses on the muscles underneath the eyes closer to the nose called musculus orbicularis occuli. These lines occur every time you squint your eyes. You may squint when looking at something bright or trying to see something close or far away. These create circles underneath the eyes, giving you a tired look.

Exercise: Place your index finger over the area where the lines start forming when you squint. Keep the fingers in place as you try to squint your eyes. You will feel the tension as your muscles underneath the eye pull closer to the bridge of your nose. Keep fingers in place and do not let them squeeze together towards the bridge of the nose.

Hold for six to ten seconds now relax the tension underneath the inside corner of your eye and let it sit back to its normal position. Keep your fingers in the same position. Breathe in more Qi and repeat the procedure.

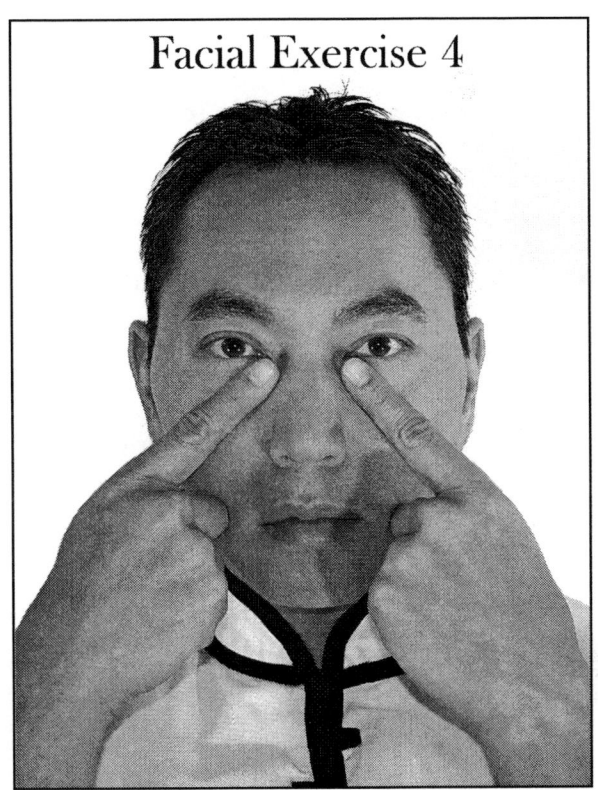

Facial Exercise 4

Perform Four Sets of six to ten repetitions with a count of six to ten seconds.

Facial Exercise 5. The fifth exercise focuses on the muscles called musculus orbicularis oris that create smile lines. These smile lines start from the bottom of each nostril and goes down to the bottom corner of the mouth. These smile lines makes your face look old and sad. They are difficult to prevent because there is a natural separation of the lip muscles from the cheek muscles, creating an invisible valley that slowly gets deeper and visible as we age.

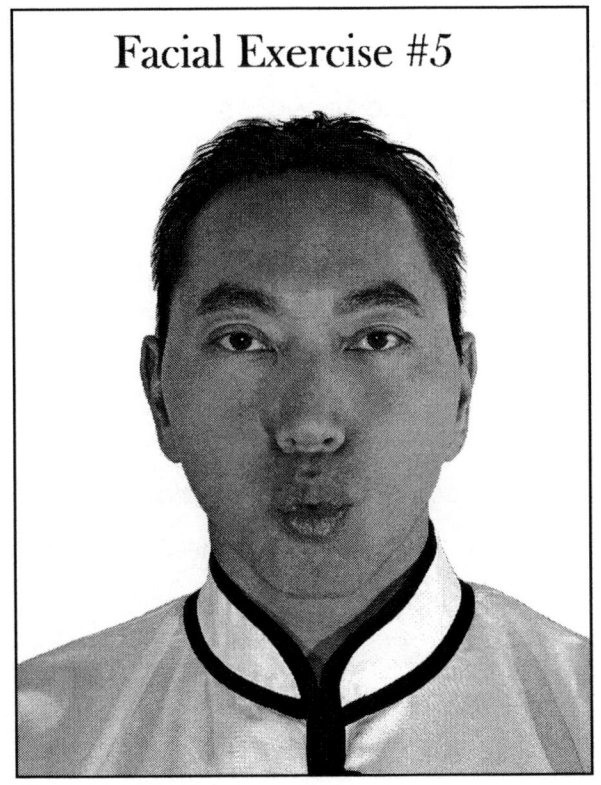

Facial Exercise #5

Exercise: Position your lips as if you were giving someone a peck on the cheek but really extend your lips as far as they will go. If you look in the mirror when you do this you will see the lip and surrounding muscles stretch to fill the natural crease of the smile line. Since you are not using your fingers on this exercise close your eyes and imagine (Yi-intention) sending Qi to this area.

Hold for a count of six to ten seconds then relax the tension and bring your lips back to its normal position. Breathe in more Qi and repeat the procedure.

Perform Four Sets of six to ten repetitions with a count of six to ten seconds.

Facial Exercise 6. The sixth facial exercise focuses on the inner lip muscles and the surrounding muscles near the lower nostril also called musculus orbicularis oris. These muscles form lines around the mouth and over time gives you that old mummy or old lady lip look or smokers lips. These tiny lines form down your upper and lower lips.

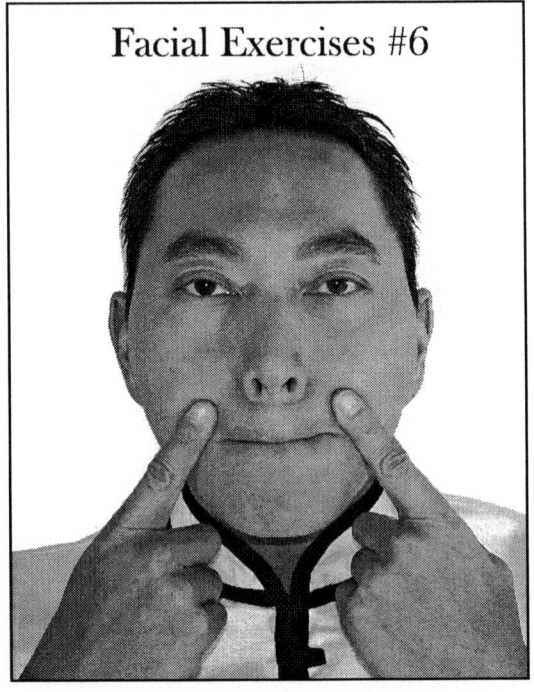

Facial Exercises #6

Exercise: Place index fingers on both sides of the corner of the mouth. This is where the corner of the mouth starts making an indentation when you smile. By placing your finger over it and pulling back slightly you prevent the indentation from forming. Now curl you lips inward as though you were hiding your lips and hold them in tightly as though trying to squeeze the two lips together. Hold for a six to ten count then relax the tension and bring the lips back to its normal position. Keep your fingers in the same position. Breathe in more Qi and repeat the procedure.

Perform Four Sets of six to ten repetitions with a count of six to ten seconds.

Facial Exercise 7. The seventh facial exercise focuses on muscles under the chin called musculus mylohyoideus. If these muscles are not toned regularly they will start to sag and you will slowly develop a double chin or what is called a turkey chin.

Exercise: Press your tongue underneath the roof of your mouth. You will feel the tension under the chin area.

Hold for count of six to ten seconds now relax the tension on the tongue and let it set back to its normal position. Breathe in more Qi and repeat the procedure.

Perform Four Sets of six to ten repetitions with a count of six to ten seconds.

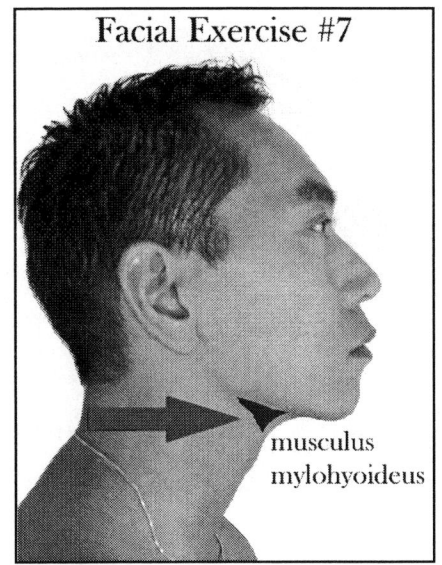

Facial Exercise #7

musculus mylohyoideus

Facial Exercise 7-b. The final Qi Gong Facial exercise is to tighten the neck and especially the jaw line muscles called musculus digastricus. Gravity tends to hold on the sides of the face creating sagging flab of skin on the jaw line and on the neck. To prevent this lie on your back. Place your head to one side and raise it. Immediately you feel your skin and muscles on the side pulling back and tightening. Again send Qi to that area that feels tight. Hold for six to ten seconds. Lower your head. Now with your head straight raise your head forward. Hold for six to ten seconds. Again you will feel the skin pull back and tension on the front of your chin and on both sides of your jaw line. In addition, you will feel tension on the front of your neck. After a count of six to ten seconds lower your head and perform the same thing to the other side of your jaw line. After doing four sets (one on each side – left side, center, right side) of six to ten repetitions for a count of six to ten seconds for each rep, you will feel the tightness on your entire jaw line and neck.

Perform my Qi Gong facial exercises at least twice a day, once in the morning and once in the evening.

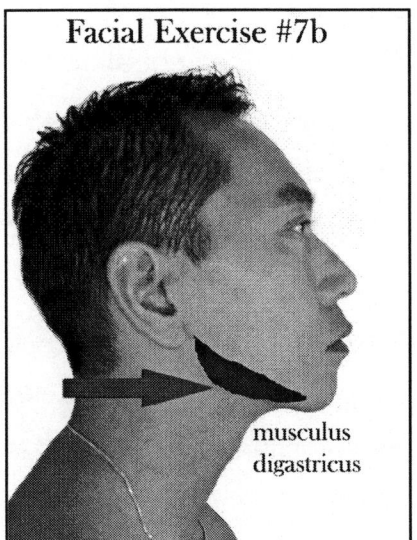

Facial Exercise #7b

musculus digastricus

Spreading the QI

After awakening the Qi you are now ready to perform my Qi Gong routine. You may begin the routine from the sitting (Egyptian or Japanese) position or standing (Qi Gong standing form) position. The Qi Gong standing form is positioning the body so that all joints, channels and meridians are not blocked. As a result the body is soft and subtle which allows Qi to flow smoothly throughout. While standing, the legs are at shoulder width and slightly bent. The back is curved in a bit at the shoulders. The head is tilted forward slightly with the chin tucked in a little bit. The arms hang over the shoulders and are bent slightly at the elbows and wrist. In the end, you look like a rag-doll with strings attached. This position insures that all the channels and meridians are free of any blockages and the body is relaxed and free of any tension. A rigid body does not allow for Qi transportation or circulation. That is why a dead body is so stiff while someone who is healthy and alive is soft and flexible.

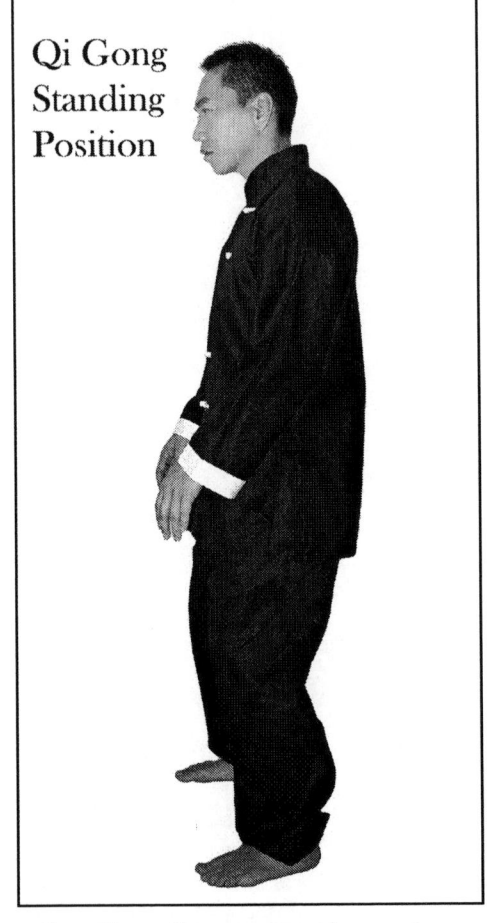

Qi Gong Standing Position

If you begin the Qi Gong routine sitting down, please be sure to be comfortable. If you are starting from the Egyptian pose please be sure to sit on the edge of the chair with the tip of your butt and make sure there is adequate cushion on the seat. The reason is that if you choose to perform the entire routine sitting down it is best that you are comfortable. Cushioning on the seat relieves pressure on your backside and lower back. Sitting on the edge of the chair makes you more aware of your position on the seat and what you are doing. In addition, if you sit too inward the edge of the chair may put too much pressure across the upper hamstring. This will start cutting some of the blood flow towards your legs and lower butt. As a result, both your legs and butt may start falling asleep (this happens when circulation is reduced in a certain area, and that tingling feeling you start to sense is when there is inadequate blood supply).

One more important thing, please choose a seat that will make your knees and butt parallel. When your knees are elevated higher than your butt the blood flow will drain from your legs as blood struggles to reach the knees and down towards the toes. As a result the area between your knees and toes will have inadequate blood circulation. However, having the knees too low puts added pressure behind the upper hamstrings on the edge of the seat therefore also cutting of blood flow.

If you are starting from the traditional Japanese sitting position proper cushioning is also stressed. With the legs folded inwards and pressure coming from the top with your own body weight it is highly possible that you will cut of blood circulation to the legs if you remain in this position for long periods. Please take caution in either sitting position (Egyptian or Japanese). The overall importance of Qi Gong exercises is letting the blood flow smoothly throughout the body; you hinder that goal through improper stance or positioning.

Relax

While sending Qi to the entire body you may say out loud a Chinese word that tells the body to relax and receive the Qi. Many other practices use chants or words like "oooommm". In this Qi Gong routine you are going to chant the word "sung"; in Chinese this means "relax". Don't forget to keep your tongue on the roof of the mouth even as you chant this word.

Spreading Qi to the entire body

Movement 1. While sitting or standing breathe in through the nose and send the breath down to the stomach. If you are performing this correctly your stomach should rise and fall with each breath. Keep doing this until you are steadily breathing through the nose and with your stomach. It is important that you are drawing in Qi adequately before you begin your routine. Not doing so will nullify any benefits you may think you are getting. In other words, you are just going through the motion without doing much. When you are ready to send Qi to each part of the body, start with the head then the neck, shoulders, back, chest, arms and finally down the legs.

Sending Qi to the head. Take a deep breath with the stomach and exhale slowly saying the word "sung" and imagine that you are sending Qi to your head. You will soon experience an amazing vibration or a light buzzing all over your head. The vibration is caused when you chant the word "sung". Because the vibration and your Yi (intention) doesn't have far to go to the head area it results in a strong sensation in your head. You will soon realize this ratio of distance to the amount of vibration sensation you feel. The further away and larger the area the less vibration of Qi you feel. That is why it is beneficial to send Qi more than once to a large area or to a body part that is further away. Once you are satisfied that you have felt the Qi vibration begin sending Qi to the next body part. Now take a deep breath with your stomach and get ready to send Qi to your neck.

Sending Qi to the neck. As you did with your head, take a deep breath and breathe with the stomach. Exhale slowly while chanting the word "sung" imagining that you are sending Qi down to your neck. Feel the vibration around your neck.

Sending Qi to the shoulders. As you did with your neck, take a deep breath with the stomach. Exhale slowly while chanting the word "sung" imagining that you are sending Qi down to your shoulders. Feel the vibration around your shoulders.

Sending Qi to the back. As you did with your shoulders, take a deep breath with the stomach. Exhale slowly while chanting the word "sung" imagining that you are sending Qi down to your back. Imagine that your back is expanding as you send Qi to that area. Feel the vibration around your back. Since the back is a large area you may not feel the vibration at first so send Qi a few more times until you do.

Sending Qi to your arms. As you did with your back, take a deep breath with the stomach. Exhale slowly while chanting the word "sung" imagining that you are sending Qi down to your arms. Feel the vibration down your arms. For some unknown reason the channels and meridians in the arms are more susceptible to experiencing Qi, allowing you to feel it more. One reason the arms are more sensitive to Qi may be because we often use the hands to send and gather Qi. In addition, we often use our hands to experience our external world and therefore may have developed a heightened sensitivity in that area.

Sending Qi to the chest area. As you did with your arms, take a deep breath with the stomach. Exhale slowly while chanting the word "sung" imagining that you are sending Qi towards the front of your chest. Like the back, your chest is a large area and therefore you may not feel the vibration of Qi as much. Send Qi to the chest area until you feel the vibration or buzzing feeling.

Sending Qi to the legs. And finally as you did with all the other body parts, take a deep breath with the stomach. Exhale slowly while chanting the word "sung" imagining that you are sending Qi down your legs and toes. Feel the vibration around the legs; however since the legs are a big body part like the back and chest, you can send Qi to each leg one at a time. In that way you can feel the vibration more.

Cultivating external Qi
near the Dan Tien

Movement 2. After sending Qi and relaxing the body you are now ready to cultivate external Qi and draw it into your body, specifically to the Dan Tien (Dantien) area. While in sitting or standing position place your palms about an inch apart just below the navel area (Dan Tien). Breathe in deeply as you start to move your hands apart about five-seven inches from each other. While breathing out slowly draw the hands together again to about one inch apart. Repeat the procedure, breathing in and out moving the palms in together (about one inch from each other) then spreading the palms away from each other (about five –seven inches).

Repetition: nine repetitions are performed

Movement 3. As with movement 2 you are doing the same moves except you are separating your hands until they are at shoulder width (Movement 3b.) and bringing them together until they are about five to eight inches apart (Movement 3a.). Repeat until nine repetitions are performed. The reason behind this is that you are trying to gather Qi around a greater area near the Dan Tien. Don't forget to breathe in as you part your hands and breathe out as you draw them closer together.

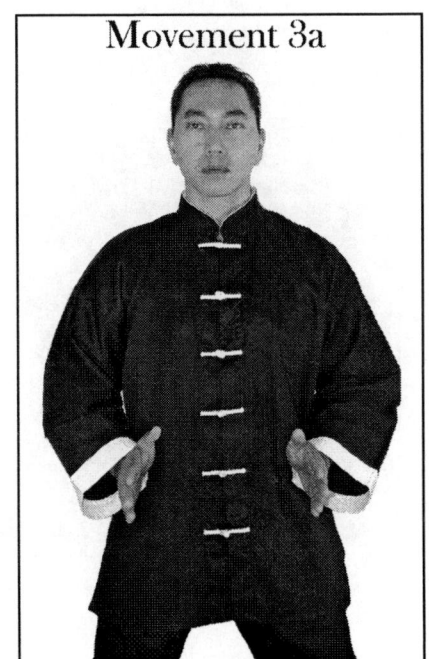
Movement 3a

Use your Yi to draw and gather Qi and always have your tongue on the roof of the mouth to complete the Micro Cosmic Orbit.

Repetition: nine repetitions

Movement 4. As with movement 3 you are doing the same thing except now when the hands are shoulder width apart imagine scooping or rounding up the Qi energy. The motion of your hands is like as though you were brushing up something, making quick scooping movements. This should be done at both sides for three repetitions. Then proceed to move the hands back together until they are about five-seven inches part and repeat the scooping movements for three repetitions.

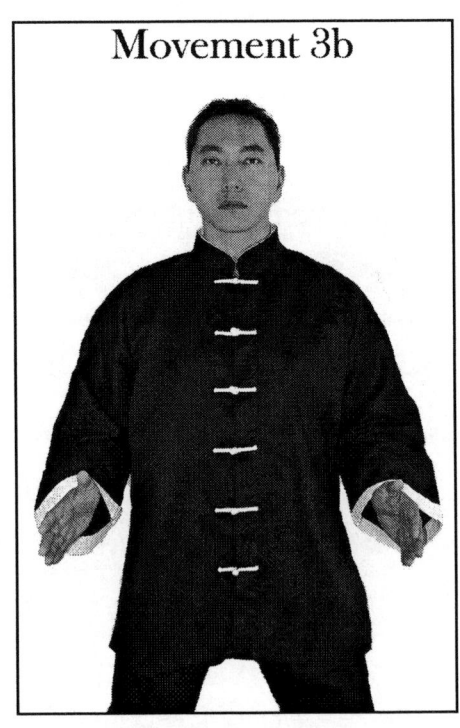

Movement 3b

This cycle of scooping Qi at the outer and inner palm locations should be counted as one repetition. Repeat until nine repetitions are performed. The reason behind this is that Movements 2 and 3 generate Qi energy around the Dan Tien and now you must gather what you have harvested.

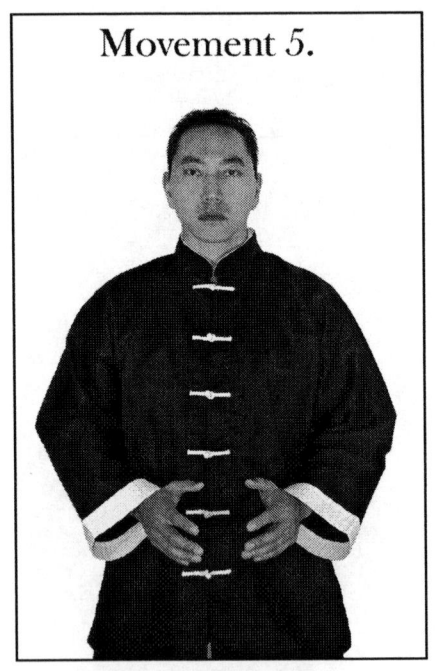

Movement 5.

Movement 5. Once you have completed Movement 4, stop with the hands about five inches apart imagining that in your hands you have gather a great deal of Qi energy. If you started the Qi Gong routine sitting you should now stand up and hold the position of your hands in front of the Dan Tien (see Movement 5.) Now imagine sending this ball of energy directly into the Dan Tien.

Cultivating Qi energy in front

Movement 6. You are now going to gather Qi energy in front of you, from your head down to the Dan Tien area. With the hands about five inches apart, breathe in deeply and move both hands up at the same time until you reach the head area (see Movement 6a, 6b, 6c). Imagine a large cylinder of Qi energy in front of you and that you are rubbing on both sides to gather up the Qi energy. Once you reach the head area start moving the hands down to the Dan Tien and then repeat for nine repetitions. Do not forget to breathe through your nose and with your stomach. Breathe in deeply as you move the hands towards the head area and exhale slowly on the way down.

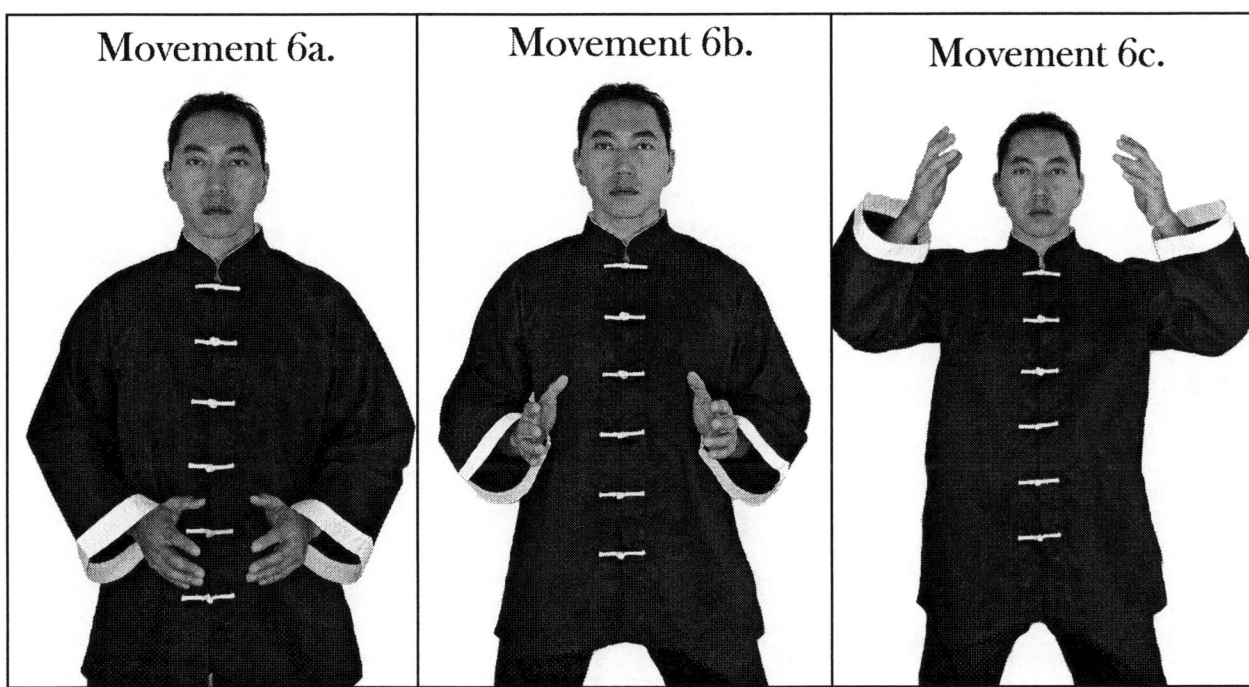

Movement 6a. Movement 6b. Movement 6c.

Movement 7. After completing movement 6 repeat the same movements but this time you will gather Qi at both the head and Dan Tien area like you did in Movement 4. Start by moving your hands upwards to the head. Once your hands are in front of your face start gathering Qi towards your face (like in movement 4, make quick scooping motions with both hands as though you are splashing your face). You are actually gathering Qi towards the Jing which is located just above the eyebrows at the center of your forehead. Jing is regarded as the Essence of Life. So by bringing more Qi towards the Jing you retard the aging process. Afterwards bring the hands down (still imagining rubbing the sides of the cylinder of energy) to the navel area and gather Qi towards the Dan Tien (as though you are splashing your lower stomach). Repeat for nine repetitions. After cultivating Qi from movement 6 you are now sending the Qi towards the Jing and Dan Tien area.

Cultivating Qi from the Earth

Movement 8. It is time to cultivate the Qi energy from the earth itself. After movement 7, spread your legs shoulder width apart and place palms facing downwards towards the floor/ground. Make circle motions in the opposite direction with each palm. Slowly move the palms outward away from the body making a circle on each side, going in opposite directions. As the palms reach the outer circle breathe in and breathe out as the palms move in towards the body completing the circle. Don't forget, your knees always follow the direction of your palms. For example as your palms move outward so do your knees; when they move inward so do your knees (see Movement 8a-8b.). Do nine repetitions for each direction when completed go to Movement 9.

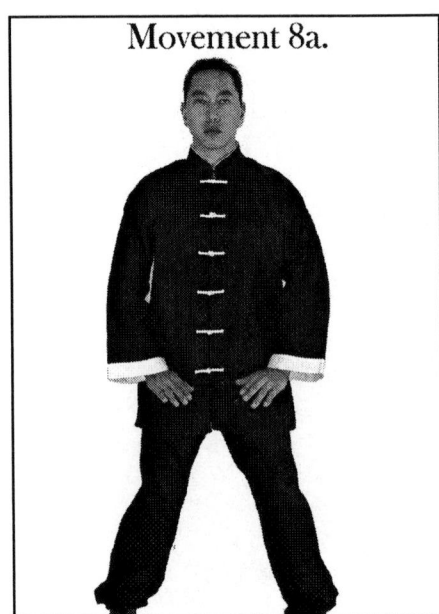
Movement 8a.

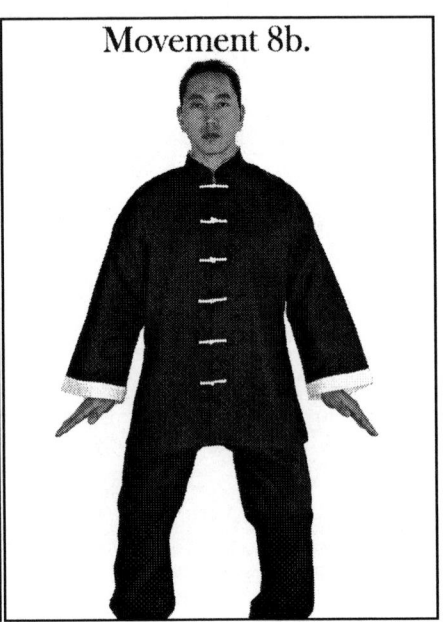
Movement 8b.

Drawing Qi into the Dan Tien

Movement 9. Bring your feet together and stand straight. With the palms of your hands make a gathering gesture to bring up the surrounding Qi in both hands. Now place both hands over the Dan Tien (just below the navel area), with the right hand over the left (see Movement 9a.). Slightly pressing on the Dan Tien area, start making small circles with your hands and then slowly making them bigger until they reach the outer edge of the Dantien (see Movement 9b –9c). Make nine rotations altogether. The last rotation, number nine, should be the biggest circle just reaching the lower chest area.

Afterwards, keeping your hands in place proceed to make another nine rotations going the opposite direction, from bigger to smaller circles. The smallest rotation should be the last one where your hands are back at the center of the Dantien.

What is happening here is that you are cultivating the Qi you have gathered from the Earth and storing it in the Dan Tien (Dantien).

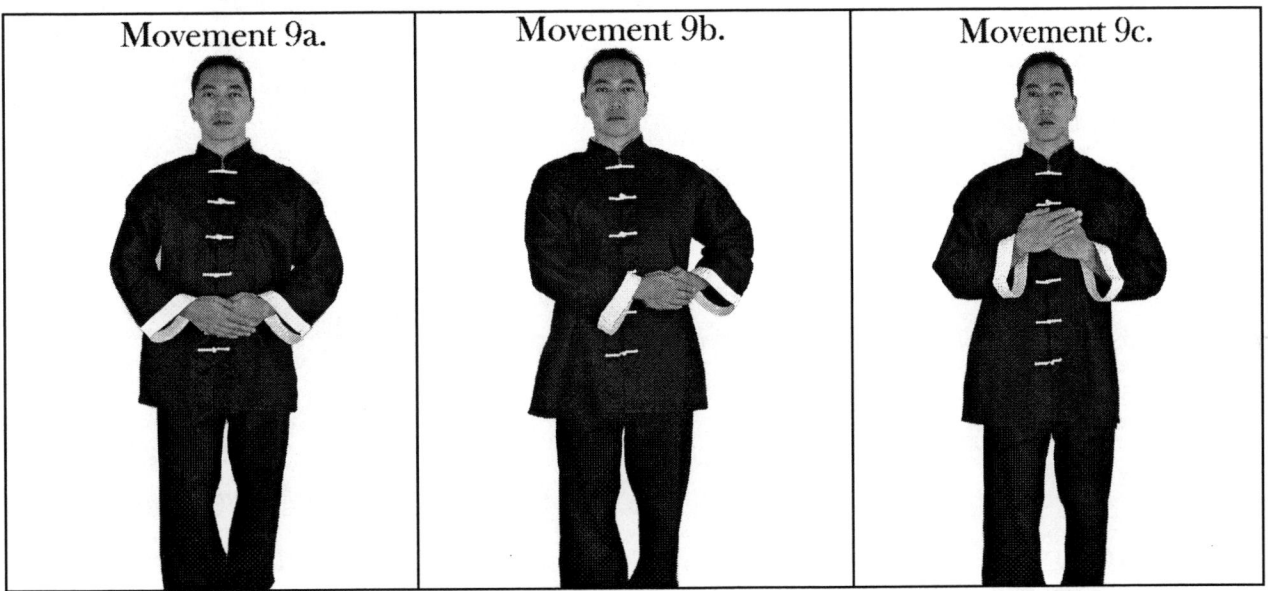

| Movement 9a. | Movement 9b. | Movement 9c. |

Cultivating Qi to the face

Movement 10. Now you will be drawing Qi up towards your face. Many practitioners notice right after Qi Gong exercises that their complexion seems clearer and their skin

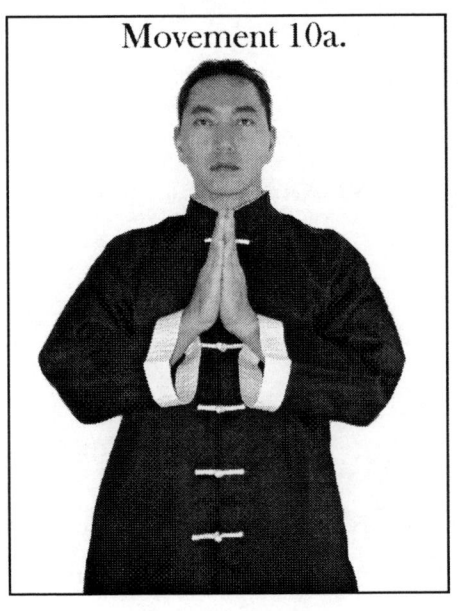

Movement 10a.

glowing; this is even more so following Qi Gong facial exercises. This is because sending Qi to the facial area, which is highly sensitive, effectively simulates the blood in that area and promotes better circulation and collagen production. Better circulation of blood in the facial area removes toxicants and creates new cells within, resulting in a fresh and glowing complexion. Begin movement 10 by bringing your hands together in a scooping motion as though you are gathering water in your hands. This movement is necessary for scooping up Qi in the Dantien and placing it on your face. Clap your hands and rub them together (Yes, that's right! just like the karate master in the movie 'The Karate Kid'). This movement simulates great amount of Qi onto your hands (see Movement 10a.). Close your eyes and imagine sending Qi energy to your hands. Keep your eyes closed and start rubbing your eyes with both hands (one hand on each eye). Rub in opposite directions for nine repetitions and then another nine times going the other way (see Movement 10b.). You are rubbing Qi directly into the eyes and the surrounding area. It is believed that this movement prevents wrinkles (lines outside the edge

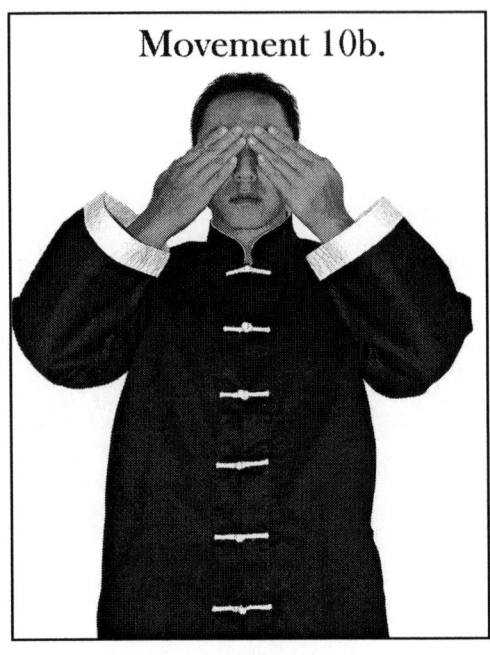

Movement 10b.

of the eyes which are called Crows Feet). In addition, movement 10 brightens eyes that are tired.

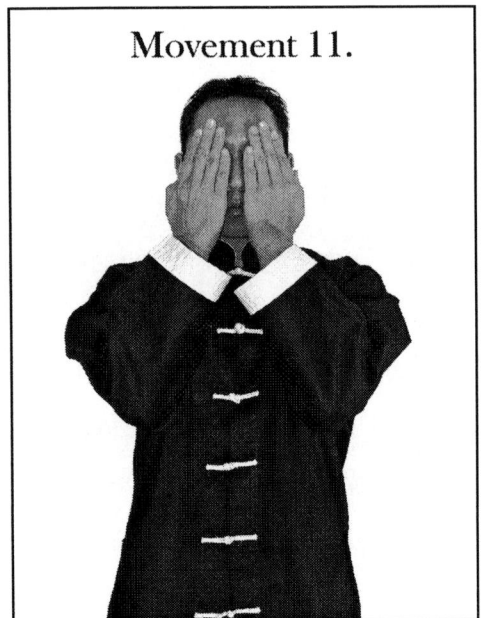

Movement 11.

Movement 11. Now that we have sent Qi into the eyes we'll now send Qi to the rest of the face. Clap your hands together again and rub them hard to generate Qi within. Place the palms of your hand on each side of your face with the pinky fingers close together. Move your hands towards the ears, imagining that you are spreading the Qi across your face. Start at the lower part of your face and with each repetition move slightly higher until you have spread the Qi to the top of your forehead. Repeat for six repetitions making sure you have spread your hands across your face evenly.

Simulating the Acupressure
points on the scalp

Movement 12. Form both of your hands into a claw-like fashion as though you are going to scratch something. Starting at the tip of your scalp, run the fingers of both hands down to the back of the neck. Repeat three times. This movement is used to simulate the pressure points on the top of your head. By simulating the scalp the Taoist sages believe it would promote healthy hair and prevent balding and grey hairs. In addition, the head has numerous acupressure points that are connected to other parts of the body like the heart. When these acupressure points are pressed they simulated these other body parts. Don't forget that you are still breathing with the stomach and that your tongue is still on the roof of your mouth (to complete the Micro Cosmic Orbit).

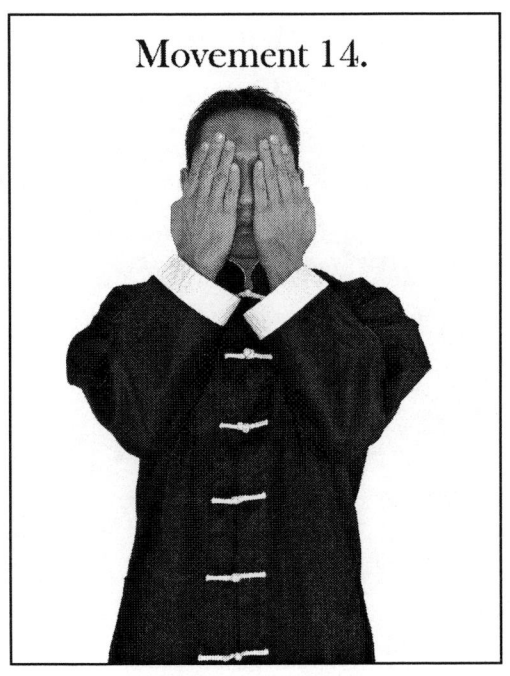

Movement 13. After running your fingers across your scalp; with the same fingers in claw-like fashion position your hands parallel to each other over the head, forming a row of four fingers across. Then like a jack-hammer, gently tap your scalp from the front to the back of the head. Again you are trying to simulate these acupressure points with your finger tips. Do three sets, with the first set beginning at the top of your head. As you progress from front to the back, tap your scalp for nine repetitions. For the second set, lower your hands slightly and again gently tap your scalp from front to back for nine repetitions. In the third and final set, place your fingers just above the ears. Gently tap your fingers on the side of your head to the back of your neck (see Movement 12).

For each row, tap your scalp for nine repetitions.

Spreading Qi to face and neck

Movement 14. Movement 14 has two steps. The first step begins after tapping your scalp with your fingers. Place the fingers of both hands on your chin; this is the starting position of Movement 14. Now run your hands parallel up over your face and head to the back of the neck. Perform the first step for three repetitions. Afterwards, the second step begins when you rub the entire face using both palms of your hands in one direction for nine repetition and then nine repetitions going the other direction. These movements circulate Qi to the entire face and head.

Movement 15. After performing movement 14 place your left hand on the Dan Tien

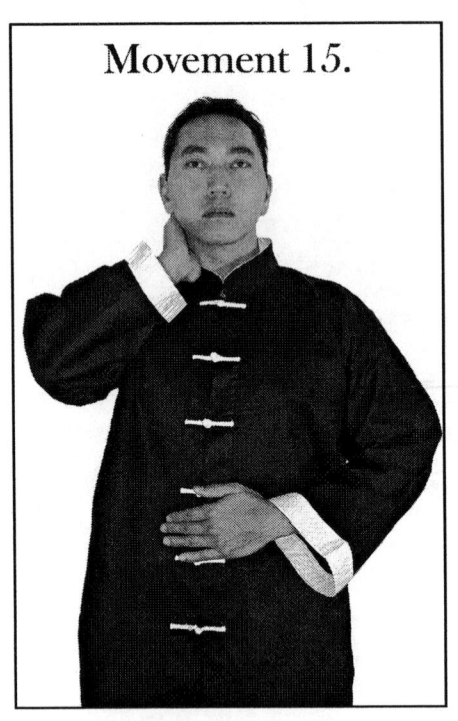

Movement 15.

(area just below the navel). With the right palm rub the right side of your neck from the front of the neck to the back for nine repetitions. Afterwards switch hands with the left hand on the left side of the neck and the right hand on the Dantien. With the left hand rub the front and back of your neck while your right hand is on the Dan Tien. This movement places Qi around the neck area by drawing up Qi energy from the Dantien. When you place your hand over the Dantien, imagine that you are drawing up Qi from that hand and transferring it to the other hand that is on either side of your neck. The reason for this is to send Qi to the sides of the neck to prevent lines from forming and keeping your neck muscles tone.

Cultivating Qi to the Dan Tien

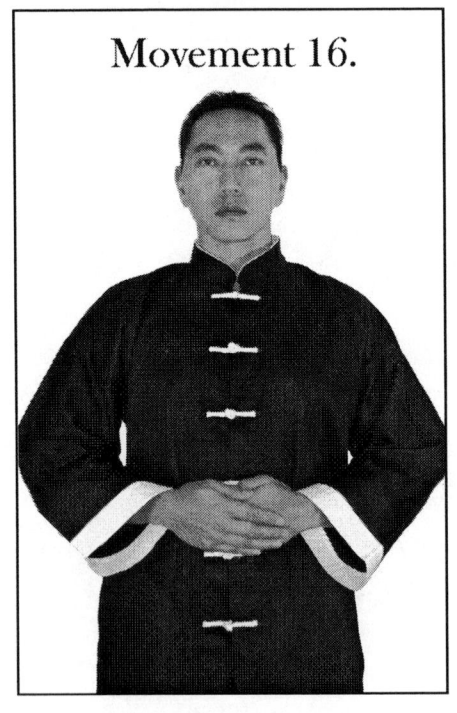

Movement 16.

Movement 16. After Movement 15 gather Qi around your navel area with your palms and place them over your Dan Tien with right hand on top. Make nine circular rotations starting with smaller ones then slowly making them bigger, like in Movement 9. Once nine repetitions are completed reverse directions for nine repetitions starting with big circles and then smaller ones until you are back to the beginning. Keep your hands where they are which should be at the centre of the Dantien, and breathe in with the stomach three times. Feel your stomach rising and falling. Say the words "Sung" as you exhale. Keep your tongue on the roof of your mouth.

Putting Qi in the mouth and creating
The Elixir of Immortality

Movement 17. This is the last movement of my Qi Gong form; you are ready to create the Elixir of Immortality by generating Qi within your mouth. There are four basic steps for creating the Elixir of Immortality. First step is to keep your eyes and mouth closed; focus on using your Yi (intention) to draw Qi towards your mouth. Secondly, gently tap together the upper and lower row of one side of your teeth making a clicking sound. Start with the right side and click your teeth together for nine repetitions. Then do the same for the left side, performing nine repetitions. Perform the same for the front teeth, for nine repetitions. Third, press your tongue on the roof of your mouth for nine repetitions. Then press the tongue on the bottom of your mouth for nine repetitions. And finally press your tongue on the back of your front teeth for nine repetitions. In the fourth step, roll your tongue inside your mouth for nine repetitions. Afterwards rotate the tongue in the opposite direction outside the teeth for nine repetitions. Keep the lips closed while doing all four steps. What is the purpose of keeping your mouth closed? The Elixir of Immortality has many forms in Taoism and one belief is that ones own saliva is the Elixir of Immortality generated from Qi movements. By keeping your mouth closed you trap the Qi that is generated within. Your saliva, otherwise known as Elixir of Immortality, that you have generated is filled with rich Qi energy that you now must swallow. As you swallow the Elixir of Immortality place your hands on the Dan Tien. Swallow a small amount of saliva and breathe in and then chant the word "sung" as you breathe out. Repeat this three times or until all the saliva has been swallowed.

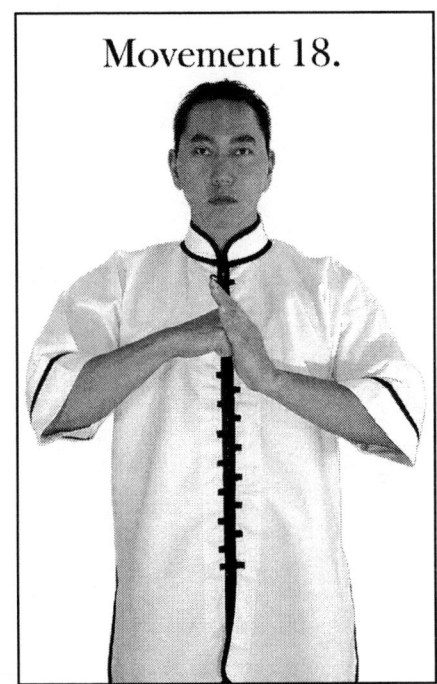

Movement 18.

Movement 18. Finish the Qi Gong routine by placing your left palm over your right fist. This is a martial arts symbol for peace and harmony. Don't forget that Qi Gong is an internal martial art specializing in the cultivation of Qi and we should always finish our Qi Gong practice with this symbol.

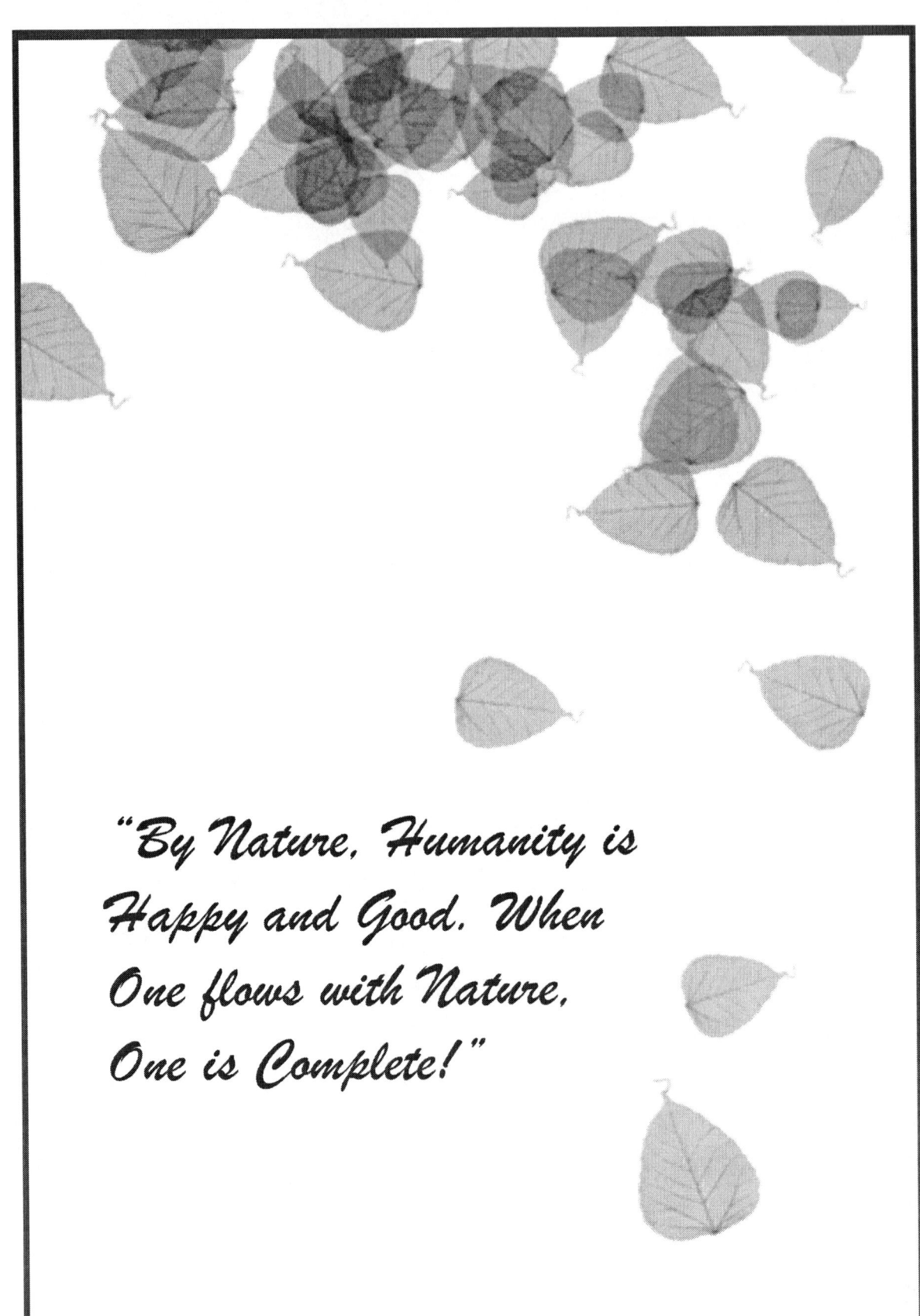

"*By Nature, Humanity is Happy and Good. When One flows with Nature, One is Complete!*"

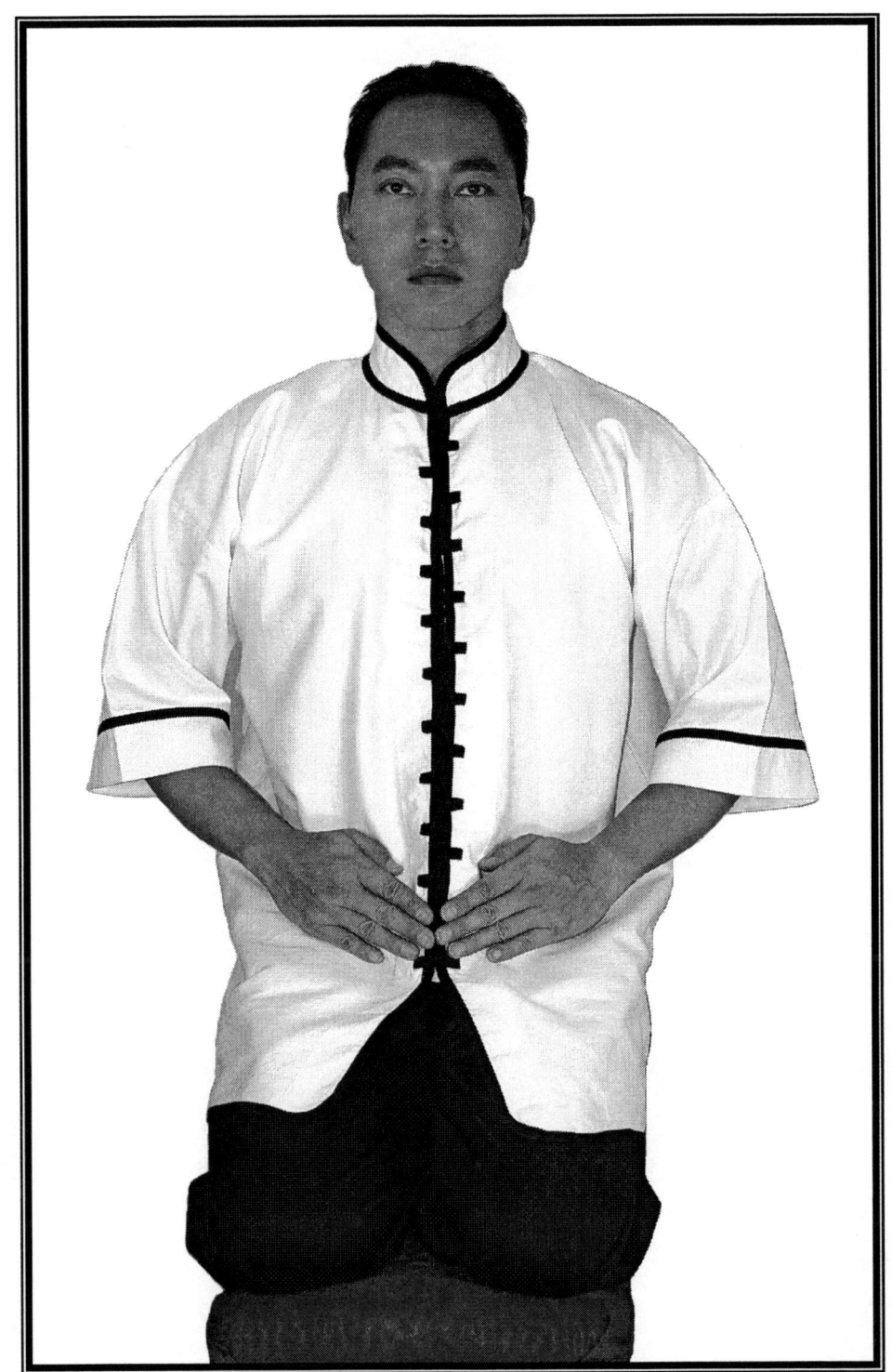

Norm Than in Sitting Meditation

More Taoist Wisdom!

"It's nice to be important… but it's more important to be nice!" N.T

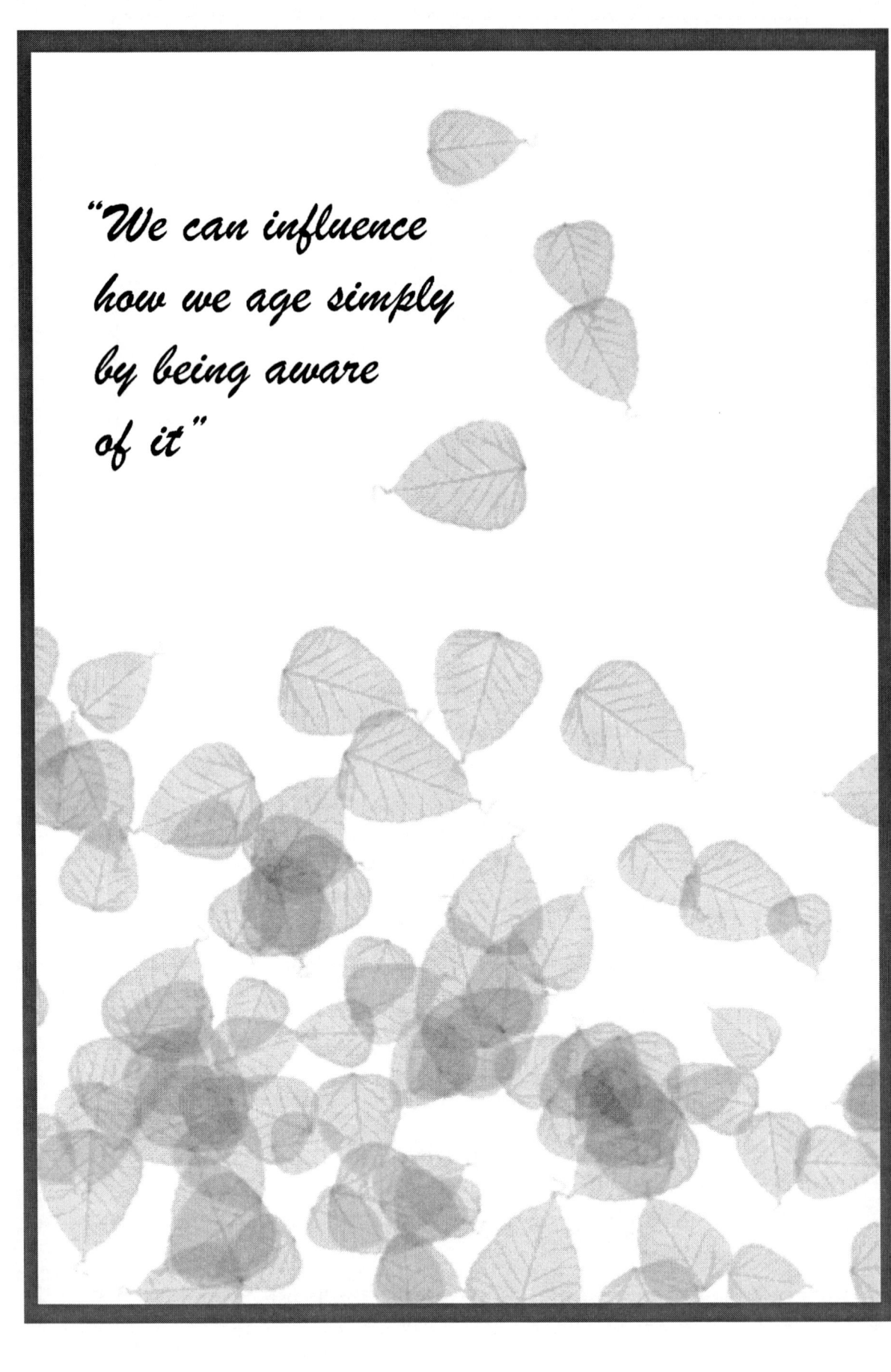

"We can influence
how we age simply
by being aware
of it"

A part of something

When a person knees and clasps their hands together and asks God for help, we say he/she is praying. But when this person hears God answering back, we say he/she is delusional. We readily dismiss the claims of others; when we don't experience the same thing ourselves. Anyone who stands out awkwardly from the crowd is not part of the group. Human beings have a primitive need for approval from their peers. This approval not only helps us become a part of society but to survive and prosper.

As you diligently practice and progress with the Three Treasures you will slowly stand out from the crowd. While your friends, family and society as a whole grow older you will not. This process will continue until you become an outcast because you are no longer part of the norm. Your friends and family complain of arthritis, grey hairs, menopause and all the other sufferings of old age but you are untouched. You are left out of social conversations because you are still young and have nothing in common with your friends who are now senior citizens. You get mistaken for someone's nephew or younger sibling and you can't even get a senior citizens discount because no one believes your true age! These situations may all be too true for the person who has dedicated his/her life to practicing the Three Treasures.

Yet another real possible scenario is watching your love ones pass away one by one until you are the last person standing, still young, healthy with years to live. These are some of the possible fears that may wait those achieving longevity. But the most worrisome situation is being alone when everyone is gone.

Loneliness

What is the point of staying young, healthy and having a long life if it turns out to be miserable? Is this why ancient sages have chosen to live in isolation in the mountains?

It is against human nature to be isolated; human beings are a social animal that needs contact with others. Being alone is a great fear and many would welcome death to end the suffering. But preserving the Three Treasures into old age doesn't guarantee that you'll be burying your friends and family and living the rest of your life in loneliness. Just because you've been practicing the Three Treasures doesn't necessary mean that you'll succeed in out living everyone else. Just like being the only member with a healthy lifestyle in a family of smokers and drinkers doesn't guarantee you'll survive and your family won't. Remember you're still mortal even if you are preserving the Three Treasures and looking like a million bucks in your old age.

Being alone is different from loneliness; many orphans and homeless people don't have families or friends but do have others who love them. A person may have a large family and many friends and still could be lonely. Being alone doesn't automatically lead to loneliness; suffering from loneliness isn't always because you're alone.

So preserving the Three Treasures will not necessarily lead to a life of solitude, nor does it require you to spend the rest of your days as a hermit. The myth of Taoist hermits living in solitude does have some fact to it. Preserving the Three Treasures does take dedication and some do seek solitude only to get away from any distraction, this however is not a requirement for achieving immortality. Preserving the Three Treasures only gives you an opportunity to stay young, healthy and to achieve longevity. What you do, who you meet, and how you live your live is up to you. You can spend it on your own or with loved ones, the choice is yours. From a Taoist point of view, we are all part of nature and connected to it physically and spiritually so we are never alone.

Death

Many fear death and try all sorts of things to keep on living. Cloning, deep freezing and expensive medical surgery are a few anti-death tactics that are used to keep one alive as long as possible. Others welcome death because they see it as the only way of escaping their present misery. For example, most old people do not fear death but what they fear is the pain and suffering that comes with old age. So in this situation they would welcome death as a permanent relief to their suffering. But the problem stems from how people perceive death. Those who fear death perceive it as an eternal end, the final existence of their lives. Those who welcome death perceive it as an escape, a crossing over to a better place. These misconceived ideas about death only make us spend the better part of our lives either fearing it or seeking it!

The Next Stage

Death comes to everyone, even to ancient sages who have lived hundreds of years. When it is time to let go of the earthly realm, the ancient sages prepare the Shen (Spirit) for the next stage or transformation. In Taoism, death is a part of living and is just a transformation that naturally takes place in the Great Tao of things (the universe).

As mentioned previously, Taoist view the world and the entire universe as composed of opposite forces (Yin and Yang) both creating and destroying, in other words in a continuous flux of transformation. It is a circle that has repeated itself since the beginning of everything. Life and death is the same thing.

If a Taoist sage who seeks immortality knows death will eventually come, why would he even bother preserving the Three Treasures?

A Taoist sage doesn't seek immortality because he is afraid of dying! The Taoist sage seeks immortality on earth to prepare their Shen (Spirit) for transformation into the Great Void. To exist in the Great Void one requires an Enlightened Spirit. Upon his death the ancient sage's body will return to the earth while his spirit continues forever. It is said that when an ordinary person dies this Spirit (Shen) leaves their body through the chest and dissipates, but an enlightened sage's spirit leaves through the top of his head and lives forever. The top of the head is believed to be the exit point to the Great Void.

Seeking the Heavens

Most people believe in some type of a Heaven or Nirvana while others may believe in karma and an afterlife or reincarnation. Even the rational and scientific minded believe there is something after death but are unsure what it is while the rest are undecided. I believe everyone is correct in some aspect on their concept of what happens after death. From a Taoist point of view, they're all partly right!

Many believe in a Paradise waiting for us after death or a continuous birth and death cycle resulting in many lives experienced. But the underlying force driving these concepts is trying to live a life well spent or a life that is meaningful so that one deserves entrance into some final divine destination. The idea of existing in a wondrous place for all eternity pushes us to follow certain religious lifestyles, perform dogmatic recitals and or acts. For example, a religious follower is expected to live by the guidelines set by their faith. These guidelines (if followed) are supposed to prepare the individual for a lifetime in Heaven. All religions have rules of conduct one must adhere to if one wishes an afterlife of peace and happiness. Others believe that we are reincarnated or reborn a number of times so we can get 'it' right. The 'it' I am referring to is living a humble and honorable life of good deeds and building enough karma to escape being reborn.

Taoism is different in several ways. First, Taoist does not believe in an All-seeing, All-knowing Supreme-being who is the creator of everything. So there is a good chance that Taoist do not believe in a Heaven as described in religious books. Taoist subscribe to the continuous transformation created by opposing forces of Yin and Yang. However, Laozi believed there was an underlying force guiding us towards a certain path and he called it our Inner Nature. I believe our Inner Nature is made from balanced Yin and Yang forces. This is why we instinctively seek a balance within ourselves, why we seek a balance with nature and why we seek a greater balance beyond our own comprehension. In the end, this is why we seek a Heaven, Nirvana or even the Great Void.

Taken with a grain of salt!

Besides standard images of angels playing harps and everyone wearing white robes and walking on white fluffy clouds, does anyone really know what Heaven will be like? Religions paint a pretty and vivid picture of Heaven and yet smear horrific and disturbing images of Hell. Since you can't have one without the other; Taoism would consider both Heaven and Hell as one of the same places. This makes sense because you wouldn't know what was good if you didn't know what was evil. What you consider evil may be viewed by others as good and vice versa. In the end, good and evil co-exist, it is how we perceive something that determines how we react, understand and believe as true. So both concepts of Heaven and Hell reside within the individual as their thoughts create the very reality that they perceive. Many ancient sages speak of 'thoughts as real and the physical body as an illusion'. We have a hard time excepting this philosophical thought because we only experience our world through our senses but yet we accept Heaven and Hell with no past knowledge of it. The power of our beliefs, our thoughts and our perceptions guide our reality. Thoughts create our reality, you control your thoughts, and therefore you control your reality!

But do you know what thoughts are? Scientist has a strong indication that thoughts are actually electrical waves. So when you think about something you are actually sending out electrical waves. Some scientists suggest that the energy produced by thoughts may explain telekinesis and ESP. When you think about something often (your dominant thoughts) your mind sends out electrical waves that go about to try and create or make happen what you have been thinking about. So if you ever had an urge of phoning someone and the phone rings with the other person on the other line; there is a good chance that your thoughts influenced the other person into thinking the same thing with you. Similar, if one's dominant thoughts are affirmatives of remaining young then one creates electrical waves that seek to create these dominant thoughts.

Some scientists have theorized that when the universe ends and collapses within itself a new life form for humanity will emerge. These new life forms will consist only of a highly evolved clustered of electrical impulses flowing around space. This new concept is not that far-fetched; since our brain functions are based on millions of electrical activity happening every second as the neuron synapses in our brain send charges between themselves. Without these electrical charges firing constantly our minds would not function, we would not have a sense of awareness.

So where does our awareness/consciousness come from? Could it be that our consciousness, awareness or enlightened spirit are created by these electrical impulses? Or are these clusters of electrical impulses actually our enlightened spirit? Maybe the mystics and ancient sages were correct, with no physical body one doesn't have to worry about primary or materialistic needs; there is no sense of greed, no awareness of good or evil and of right or wrong. Could it be that these clusters of electrical impulses are what the mystics and Taoist sages spoke of! Could they be the last evolutionary phase of humanity?

A vision of loveliness

Most people associate degenerative eyesight with old age, but these problems also happen to young people so this association is false. Most people do not know that the main reason we lose some of our eyesight capabilities is because 1) we abuse our eyes, 2) we don't exercise them enough and 3), we rather keep wearing glasses which really doesn't help and makes them worst in the end.

There are many ways in which we abuse or hinder our eyesight. One of them is prolong exposure to the TV or computer screen. Sitting in a darken room staring at the bright lights from the television for hours at a time strains the eyes. We try to recreate a cinema atmosphere by turning all the surrounding lights off and having one central light coming from the TV. We think by focusing all the light on the TV that we get a better image and it is easier on our eyes and it helps us concentrate on what's going on. Instead this strains the retinas by letting in too much concentrated light at the one time. It is like staring directly at the sun which we now know can damage or even blind you. Yet we do the same thing with our television set, only we are doing it less intensively but over a long period of time the effects are the same. We can do ourselves a favor and turn on some lights to reduce the glare from the TV which puts less strain on our eyes.

Secondly, we let our eyes get out of shape by not exercising them on a regular basis. Yes, that's right exercise for the eyes. If this is the first time you have heard of this I am not surprised. Millions of people have not heard of exercising the eyes to improve eyesight mainly because most of us believe it is out of our control. It is hard to imagine performing eye exercises like push-ups for the arms and chest. The American Vision Institute is the best source to get information on eye exercises to improve and correct the most simple vision problems like near and far-sightedness. The reason most people have not heard of such a thing is because the medical and optometry fields do not recognize its importance or nor do they bother to inform their patients about them. Again this is not surprising because most optometrist will be losing patients if everyone had the ability and know-how to improve their vision themselves. If you were an optometrist with a thriving business would you let your clients know that instead of buying expensive glasses and depending on them for the rest of your life you can easily improve your vision safely and permanently by doing a few simple eye exercises? Of course not! If you think there is a battle going on between institutes like AVI and optometry colleges you are correct. But eye exercises only improve and correct eyesight problems that are correctable, meaning problems that do not require surgery. Implementing eye exercises as part of the overall health care by optometrists would be beneficial for all those concerned.

The main reason for eye exercises is that it is believe that we have forgotten how to use our eye muscles; in other words we got lazy. Let me explain, for example when there is something at the corner of our eyes we should simply move our eyes to that corner to see what is it. But instead, we actually turn our whole head around to face it directly and to view it. This is because it is easier to turn the whole head resulting in less strain than looking out at the corner of your eyes. The problem is we don't let our eye muscles do the work. By making it easier on the eye muscles we actually forced them out of shape. It is like getting a really powerful lens for your camera and only using one setting and ignoring all the zoom capabilities and wide angle options. Or driving a manual car and only using one gear. The other gears need to be used or they will get rusty and the one gear that is overworked will get weaker and weaker until it breaks down. Your eyes are the same and you need to use all ranges of your eyesight to keep them in tip top shape. Here are a couple of eye exercises that you can do anywhere. Eye Exercise 1. Take hold of a pen and place the end of it about six inches away from your eyes. Look at the tip or end of the pen and pay attention to the details. Now keeping your eyes on the pen start moving it further away from your eyes with your hand until your hand is at arms length. While the pen or pencil is moving further away keep focusing on the fine details until the pen is at arms length. Then bring the pen back slowly and again keep your eyes peeled on the tip or end of the pen. Move the pen up toward your face until it is six inches away from your eyes. Notice the slight strain on your eyes when you paid close attention to the details of the pen and again when the pen was moved further back and then closer. When you were adjusting the focus with your eyes you were actually exercising the retinal muscles.

Eye Exercise 2. Find an object that is in front of you, then find another one a little further away and then find one that is at a distance. Without moving take turns focusing on details of each object. First the object closest to you then the object further away and then the farthest object. Keep focusing and rotating from object to object. When the furthest object becomes clearer with practice move it a couple of feet back and repeat the entire exercise. This will force your retinal muscles to adjust (strengthen) to the new length and therefore increase the distance of your eyesight.

There are a lot more different eye exercises one can do. It is best to contact the American Vision Institute to find out more information about exercises for your eyes.

Even the ancient Taoist ages recognized the need to care for ones eyes and have devised Qi Gong exercises to send Qi directly into the eyes to strengthen it. One Qi Gong method was to send Qi directly to the finger tips and then rub the eyes. One would imagine rubbing the Qi directly into the eyes and strengthening them. They also realized that continuous straining of the eyes and prolong exposure to light was damaging to the eyes and often gave them a 'rest' through meditation, or going into the shade or soaking them in a bowl of clean warm water.

Third, we think we are aiding our eyes by wearing prescription glasses but we are actually making them weaker. For example, you have broken your leg and have to use crutches to aid in your walking. After your leg is fully healed you still use the crutches to aid in your walking. Sounds a little odd doesn't it? but you are doing the same thing wearing glasses. Eyewear only reinforces your dependence on them. You will constantly need stronger prescription as your eyesight gets weaker!

Drugs, It's not just for kids anymore!

I am not a big fan of taking prescribed medical drugs for ailments that could be remedied through alternative means. More often than not, medical drugs are prescribed for simple illnesses. As a result, doctors and many pharmaceutical companies together cohort a never ending dependence from the very people they're suppose to help. This growing dependence has become a billion dollar industry and has created a drug monopoly that only caters to those who could afford them.

Many of the giant pharmaceutical companies have millions invested in the sale of drugs for seniors and society as a whole. Doctors are encouraged to prescribe drugs to their patients. But patients are also to blame. For example, many visit their doctor expecting to be given something to cure them. Surprising, few are satisfied with a report indicating that nothing is wrong with them. When one pays thousands for an MRI report, they expect to see something wrong. In other words, patients themselves create this imaginary need for more prescription medicines which the doctors and drug companies are only too eager to satisfy.

In the most industrialized countries, there is no such thing as health care but only 'sick' care. Millions are prescribed drugs they don't even need, making patients worst of and more depended on the drugs. The listed side affects of the drugs are as bad as the illness itself. Unfortunately, In the end it is all about money. New drugs will always be created to meet the never ending demand to relieve simple discomforts. For example, there are at least ten different brands of medicine offering relieve for the same ailment.

There are many well written books on this subject but the main point from a Taoist view is 'let the body cure itself'. For the ancient sages, there is an antithesis for all ailments, weather through Qi movement, acupuncture or herbal remedies. Most illnesses and ailments can be cure through safer alternative means. In the East one would never prescribe to taking drugs to cure an ailment unless all natural and alternative medications have been tried. From a Taoist point of view, one reason mankind seems to be suffering from more illnesses is because he is not exposing himself to the natural elements of nature. For example allergies and hay fever are the result of an immune system that has been confined and has never experienced different types of viruses before. Case in point, a country boy would not likely be allergic to animal hair whereas a boy who was confined to the city would.

Fortunately, in the West there is now a movement to homeopathic and natural medicines and ancient Chinese practices such as acupuncture are becoming popular. Surprisingly, the force behind this movement are medical professionals themselves who, in the wake of losing patients to alternative therapies, have regulated patients to seeing only medical doctors who are qualified in TCM (Traditional Chinese Medicine). This is a sneaky way of recuperating patients lost to alternative medicine practitioners. Remember, it is all about money not what is best for the patient!

Medical Science
and the Fountain of Youth

Medical science has come a long way in improving the quality of human life. But all attempts to find the Fountain of Youth has ended in disaster. Ancient Chinese rulers wanted to gain immortality and sought mystics and masters of herbal remedies. They drank poisonous mixtures that contained mercury and other deadly concoctions which either made them seriously ill or caused certain death. For centuries and till this day, mankind has searched for a magic potion that will give him everlasting life and still there is no safe shortcut to the Fountain of Youth except for practicing the Three Treasures. Growth hormones injected into the body revitalized certain parts of the body for a short period of time but in the long run will lead to certain consequences such as cancer and heart problems. When mankind thinks they have found a shortcut to restoring youth and health it always leads to more problems. From a Taoist point of view, the only safe and surest route to longevity is to have a healthy lifestyle and preserving the Three Treasures.

I already have an active lifestyle and a healthy eating habit, why do I need to preserve the Three Treasures?

Good question! Time is always against us. We all grow older and that's what aging is and that's called being alive. Being physically active with good living habits improves your chances of a long healthy life but there are no guarantees except one – you will die someday, it is up to you weather you want a short or long life. The Qi within your body naturally flows through the meridians or channels of the body, keeping it healthy and mobile. Even the most health conscious person needs to move his/her Qi throughout the body to stay alive. When the Qi is not moving then sickness and death occurs even to the fittest of individual. Stories of fit individuals suffering from freak heart attacks or illnesses are actually the result of Nature of Chaos. Nature of Chaos is actually an event within nature that randomly occurs. However, combining a healthy lifestyle and preserving the Three Treasures reduces the chances of Nature of Chaos occurring within us and helps in achieving longevity.

A Super Model Diet

Scientific/medical labs have experimented on extreme diets to prolong life and found that a strict calorie-reduction diet can increase ones lifespan. It has been proven in medical labs with lower form animals such as mice and rats and even insects (fleas). It is a very rigorous, if not potentially fatal, regiment of diet that pushes one close to starvation. The main theory is that if the body was thinking it was starving or in danger of malnutrition the immune system slows down to conserve energy and moves nutrients to feed only the main organs, heart, brain and lungs. As a result everything slows down even aging. This type of diet is potentially life threatening. It constantly stresses the body by making it think it is in danger (starvation). The more stress on the individual the more they age so therefore this diet is self defeating.

The Taoist, however, did see value in restricting the body of food from time to time but only for very short durations. One method the Taoist used to restrict calorie intake was fasting. The Taoist were not the only ones who saw the value of fasting, many other religions perform the same practice. Fasting takes form in different ways. For example there is juice fasting where the practitioner drinks only juices from vegetables or fruits. Another Taoist fasting method is not eating and only drinking water for two days. In the end, fasting gives the stomach a chance to recuperate and the body time to cleanse and to use up stored energy within the body. The body naturally keeps energy reserves in case of famine or for fight or flight emergencies. So fasting is both a chance to rest the stomach and to burn off those fat cells.

Under the knife

Why should I spend so much time practicing the Three Treasures to stay young and healthy and achieve longevity when plastic surgery gives the same results but quicker?

It looks like everyone is getting something done to their body features that they don't like or want to improve. More surgeons, cheaper prices and a population hung up on looks and a need for approval has led to an artificial society. It's not just the movie stars who are getting something done to improve their looks, its housewives, men, high school students and anyone who can afford it. Once a taboo and kept a secret now many gladly tell all about what type of plastic surgery they had done recently to anyone who would listen. So why practice the Three Treasures when a day under the knife can have you looking younger now? Well, there is a reason why they call it 'plastic' surgery. The word plastic means artificial, fake or not real. So plastic surgery is in hence, a synthetic version of the real person.

There is no doubting the amazing results of plastic surgery but cultivating the Three Treasures will promote a younger, healthier you which, hopefully, that will last longer than your plastic surgery. The Three Treasures should not be looked upon as a replacement for plastic surgery but as an additional treatment in keeping you looking your best. Supposed you just had a facelift that made you look five years younger (I would caution to say no more than that!). Practicing my Qi Gong facial exercises will aid in keeping your new look a bit longer; just like a healthy diet and physical training will help you maintain the results you received from your tummy-tuck operation. Without taking care of yourself the results you received from your plastic surgery will not last. Facial expressions, poor eating habits, gravity (yeah, gravity!) has a way of making a new improved body looking old and wrinkle in a few years.

Longevity tests

Years ago the medical science field wanted to find the answers to why and when humans start aging? Longevity tests were developed to identify possible traits or characteristics for long life. They studied individuals who had lived a relatively long life and tried to see if there were similar traits amongst them. The results showed that satisfaction at work, marriage and family life played a major role to aging well. Whereas smoking, drinking and being non-active sped up aging. These results proved little since the oldest individuals in the study did not work, were not married, drank and smoked on occasions and were alone most of their lives. The problem with medical/scientific tests is that they only see facts and variables that could be identified. Scientists will never be able to categorize the whole process of aging because there are too many mixtures of variables, some seen and others hidden. These studies only give medical science a clue to longevity and therefore offer a misconception of aging as a whole.

The Hayflick experiment vs. Three Treasures

Another medical/scientific experiment has resulted in the famous Hayflick experiment, which had shown that human cells have a limited amount of times they can divide (grow or expand) before the cell reaches its capacity and starts dying. Therefore, humans in theory can only live till a certain age before they start dying (aging). However, the original Hayflick results incorrectly showed that human cells divided infinitely. This was because Prof. Hayflick who tested chicken cells in a pantry dish accidentally kept feeding the cells and they keep on dividing. Fortunately, other laboratory tests to back Hayflicks' claim showed that both chicken cells and human cells do have a maximum growth cycle (max. amount of times they can divide) before they start dying. While other tests showed that humans could not live forever it was the Hayflick experiment which initially started the whole process of testing for human aging.

These tests are significant in my theory of how the Three Treasures have worked for me and the path to Youthful Immortality that I want to achieve. I believe that through Qi movement one can 1) keep cells healthy and vigorous and 2) at the same time produce new and stronger cells to replace the cells that could not divide anymore and have died. This balance I believe can be obtained through the continuing restoration and development of the Three Treasures. So in my humble opinion it is better to start the practice of the 3Ts at a relatively young age as I did. In theory, once you have reached your peak maturity (the max. amount your cells can divide) you start to age (the cells start dying). For example, imagine your life as a roller coaster ride which is at the top (your cells can't divide anymore) and now you are heading downwards (you age) and there is nothing you can do about it (nature at work). If you mastered the 3Ts at a young age (before the roller coaster reached the top) for example in my case at the age twenty-three, you should be able to slow down or even stop the coaster from reaching the top and going down. So in theory I have been able to stop the descent of the coaster and remain living at my peak through the practice of the 3Ts. Presently I believe my cells are kept healthy and vigorous while old and dead cells are replaced with the movement of my Qi. Look at the chart below as it theorizes the process of an individual starting the 3Ts when they are a young adult. The top chart shows the normal progress without practicing the 3Ts. The bottom chart shows the progress of the 3Ts as one would look like till old age.

Child – Adolescent – Young Adult - Mature Adult - Middle Age – Golden Years

Start 3Ts

Child – Adolescent – **Young Adult --Young Adult ---Young Adult – Young Adult**

This is not saying that it is too late to start practicing 3Ts if you are middle aged or in your golden years, the 3Ts will work at any age. On the other hand, it is very difficult (but not entirely impossible) to slow down or stop a roller coaster when it is speeding downwards as compared to when it is slowly climbing upwards. Conscientiously starting the 3Ts at a later stage in your life will not make you young again but it will certainly slow down your aging if you let it.

It isn't just the medical world that is keeping us old; it is our society. From his best selling book, "Ageless Body, Timeless Mind", Deepak Chopra points out that aging is something that society through social conditioning has taught our bodies to do. Through our society we have learned how to age. And what we learned has turned into a core belief. Our beliefs about aging are stronger and deeper than rational and reasonable thoughts. In other words, we age because we give in to rigid assumptions and beliefs. As Deepak Chopra states we hold on to our beliefs because we think they are true. Not even hard evidence or logical conclusion disproving our beliefs would change our minds. That is why using rational thought processes tend not work with people with phobias because their rational thoughts are overridden or clouded by their beliefs. Beliefs have in some respect turned into something that represents the individual and giving it up would be like losing part of themselves and that is why they have such power over us. In order to change our beliefs we have to unlearn all the social conditioning that have led to our beliefs about aging. Since aging is something we learnt we actually have control to unlearn it. We do this by adopting new beliefs. Make no mistake, because your old beliefs took a lifetime to adopt and learn it will take you just as long to unlearn them and adopt new ones.

Another way we can unlearn something is by being open minded to new possibilities and opportunities and having the courage to try and change. You can start adopting and being open-minded to the Three Treasures by simply being more aware of yourself and listening to your mind and body and your Inner Nature.

Current medical breakthroughs offer a narrow alleyway to limited longevity. However, the surest pathway to immortality is one of the oldest and most traveled roads created by the ancient Taoist sages. It is safe and well-lit through the teaching of the Three Treasures. It is open to anyone willing learn from their past to change the present and to live for the future.

Human Diseases

Qi Gong against human diseases

A lot of material has been written on the affects of Qi Gong on many of humanity's illnesses, like cancer and other incurable diseases. This book is not about using Qi Gong to cure any ailments. Qi Gong does promote superior health because it influences better blood circulation. I do not claim that Qi Gong will rid your cancer or any life-threatening ailments you may have. The effects of Qi Gong on your own Qi are a personal one. Just like you have your own Tao or path to follow your Qi will work differently for you. There is no hard rule that ones own Qi will do this or that, contrary to reports written about the effects of Qi. These reports are personal accounts of other individual experiences with Qi. They are without credibility and some are just too far fetch to believe. Like the Great Tao or the tao of one's own Qi energy it is impossible to fully understand yet measure. The most honest and accurate measurement of your Qi is you! You don't have to prove your Qi to anyone but yourself. But if you practice the Three Treasures rigorously and cultivate as much Qi as you can, then you will give yourself the best chance of enhancing your immune system to fight illnesses and achieving longevity.

External Qi transferred to another person is impossible to test or detect. There have been many laboratory experiments to detect and measure Qi and few if any, were successful. People interested in proving the existence and the transfer of Qi seek valid evidence to back their claim. They are trying to give Qi and Qi Gong credibility in the eyes of Western science. The practice of Qi cultivation has been around at least three thousand years before western medicine had begun to take root. Far Eastern practices like Qi Gong should not have to seek approval from the new kid in the block in the existence of Qi. By trying to validate Qi we give more power to Western medicine.

The practice of Qi Gong is very dear and personal to me. It has given me my youth, strength and energy and has guided me throughout me life. I hate to see Qi Gong made a mockery by others claiming this and that while trying to build a name for themselves. Because the existence of Qi is hard to prove, many claim to have Qi powers or abilities in order to take advantage of the weak, desperate and gullible. It is advisable to study under a teacher or someone who has practiced Qi Gong for many years but only as a guide. It is also advisable to study under someone who is humble and at peace with themselves. These types of individuals won't let their egos or pride stand in the way in guiding others. Remember, Qi has no master and those who claim this understand less about Qi than the students they teach. The best and only Qi master is you. The best measurement of Qi success is you. The only one who can detect your Qi is you. The only one who can give you better health, youth and longevity is… you!

Cancerous Cells

Cancerous cells are created by our own body. It is not like we can catch cancer cells accidentally from someone else. There is a reason why our body creates them! So if our body can create these cells it can also destroy them as well. Since you are the master of your own body it is up to you and you alone. People claiming the ability to transfer Qi energy to destroy your cancer cells are only trying to take advantage of you. When they wave their hands in the air as though they are sending Qi to you, it is actually you who is sending Qi to the cancerous cells and destroying them. The power of the mind and Yi (intention) should not be underestimated.

When our body's Yin and Yang forces are off balance illness occurs. These illnesses are signals telling you something is wrong within you and that you should do something about it. Many will ignore these signals until it is too late when more drastic measures are needed such as surgery. It is foolish and unfair to believe that by abruptly practicing Qi Gong, one will rid themselves of serious affliction, especially when one is a novice. But desperate times calls for desperate measures! And here lies the problem. Qi Gong's real power is maintenance and balancing the body in harmony with nature, and it takes time to do that. Since your cancerous cells did not appear over night (it takes a long time for cancerous cells to develop) it is reasonable to say that it will take a while for our bodies learn to fight back!

Stress kills!

As mentioned previously, our bodies create cancerous cells and other destructive cells because of a constant imbalance of the body. From a Taoist point of view, illness arises when we are not in balance according to nature. On a daily basis many things throw us off balance and the main culprit is… STRESS! Many of the Taoist philosophies hidden agenda is to reduce stress. Unnatural desires, being materialistic, envy, jealousy etc. all create unwanted stress. Nothing ages the body or causes more illnesses than stress, in fact stress kills! But one can learn to adapt to stress and survive its attacks. For example when one is in balance with nature their wellness level may look like chart 1. When this person encounters a stressful situation their wellness chart may look like chart 2. But after the stressful situation the person returns to normal, see chart 3.

(at rest)	(stress)	(at rest)
Chart 1.	Chart 2.	Chart 3.
_____	\\\\\\\\	_____
_____	\\\\\\\\	_____

If a person doesn't learn to adapt to stressful situations they constantly put the body at some level of stress causing an imbalance, even at rest. (see charts below)

(at rest)	(stress)	(at rest)
Chart 4.	Chart 5.	Chart 6.
________	\\\\\\\\	______
________	\\\\\\\\	_____

When the body is stressed its natural reaction is to produce chemicals to counteract the imbalance. But when the body is in constant stress (see chart 4 and 6), meaning out of balance a majority of the time, then serious illness will occur because of the body's natural reaction to counteract this imbalance. The paradox is that in order to save itself the body actually starts killing itself. Cancerous cells and ulcers are signs from the body that all is not well… so start listening!

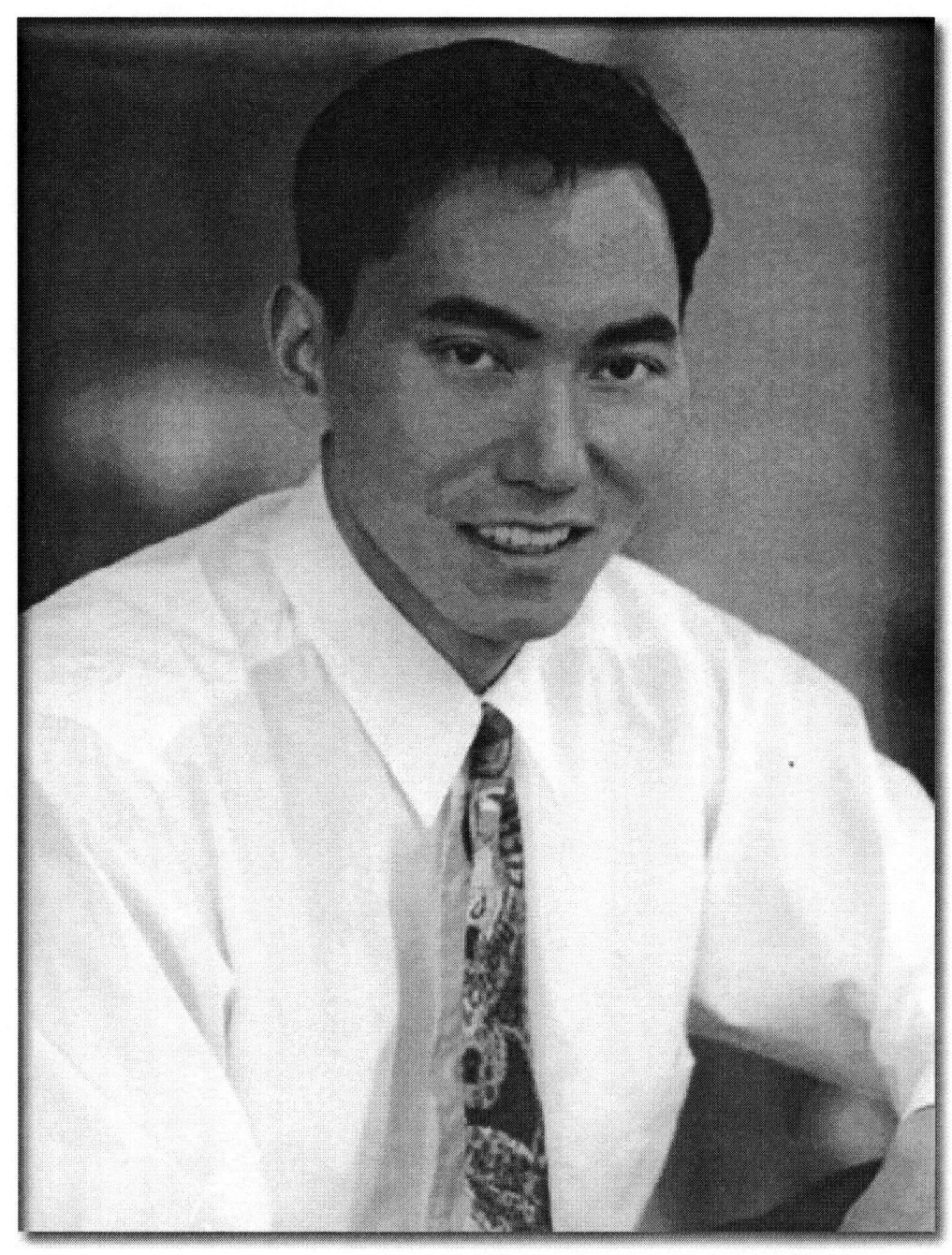

Norm Than at age 34

Sex! ...And other things

"If I added all the orgasms I had so far, it would be the best hour of my life" N.T

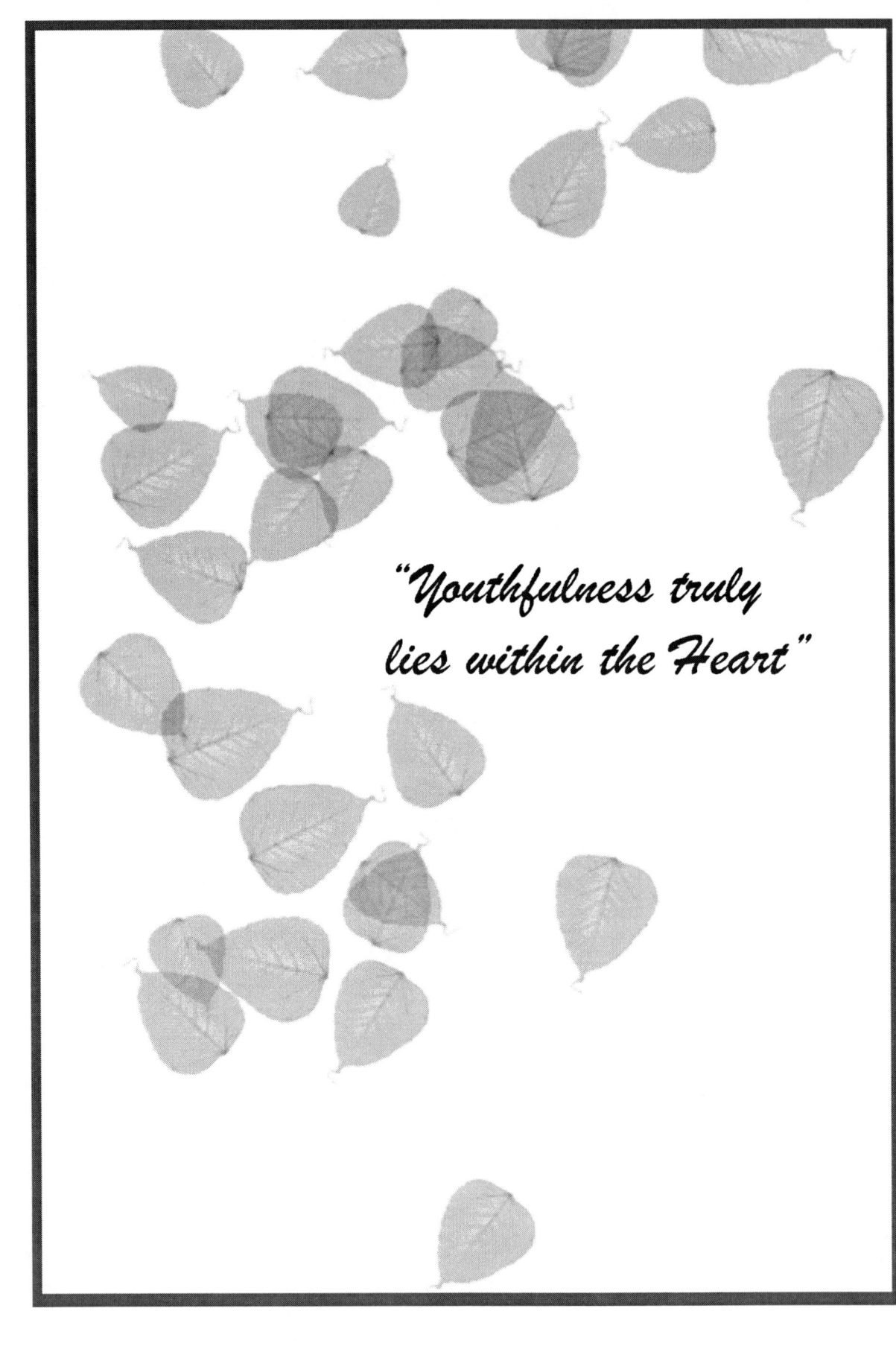

"Youthfulness truly lies within the Heart"

Sex... and other things

You sexy thing!

Now we get to the good stuff about Taoism... Sex! Taoism believes that sex is healthy and follows the Tao of nature; so one should have it often (safe sex, of course!). Most people get the wrong idea about ancient Taoist sages; that they had to give up sex in exchange for immortality. If an ancient Taoist sage was around today he would say, "Are you nuts?!" What is the point of achieving longevity or maybe immortality just to deny yourself the most pleasurable gift of nature?

But Taoism does stress that when a man loses sperm without procreation, it is a waste. This is because a lot of the body's energy goes into reproducing sperm. This energy can best be used for other productive goals. So the main idea is that sex is healthy and one should have it often but not lose any sperm through ejaculation. This sounds pretty tricky, doesn't it? To overcome this problem Taoist sages have developed sexual practices that would enable a man to 1) achieve an orgasm without ejaculation and without losing his erection 2) while at the same time heightening sexual Qi energy.

Taoist Sexual Practices

Most books about Taoist sexual practices believe that by using sexual exercises a man can achieve multiple orgasms without ejaculation and without losing his erection. In theory by performing these sex exercises the male can make love all night which is a dream come true for all men and every woman's fantasy.

I only believe part of the Taoist sexual practices. While exchanging Qi energy with a partner is doable and will heighten Qi levels in one another; I do not believe that you can separate orgasm from ejaculation. This is like having the Yang without the Yin. It is more wishful thinking than fact. Just because there are a number of books on the subject and numerous so-call sex experts have outlined instructional manuals on it; that still doesn't make it possible. A lot of men have written in to give testaments that they can achieve this practice but it is more so for their egos and something to brag about with the boys. I believe it's an ideal sexual fantasy easily believed by men. To be able to have an orgasm without losing your erection and to be able to make love all night seems too good to be true. And that's because it is. For the millions of men who dream of achieving this, the only sure way is using Viagra! A lot of men with erectile dysfunction and premature ejaculation have used Viagra to overcome this problem with a high success rate. But there are reports of complications using Viagra such heart attacks. One possible reason for heart complications is that Viagra redirects the flow of blood from other areas of the body to the genitals thereby forcing an erection. But the problem of premature ejaculation still exists; only now they're stuck with an erect penis while the body is drained of energy after orgasm. The male may as well make the best of it and use his erection as a temporary coat hanger till the formula wears out!

Taoist sexual practices include switching your concentration from love making to breathing and finger positioning to stop premature ejaculation. The problem is that while performing this act erection is lost immediately because the man's attention isn't on sex anymore. And besides these sexual practices are not practical in the bedroom, requiring the man to stop making love at full throttle and perform his sex exercises to just prevent premature ejaculation. Your partner will be disappointed and will also be wondering what the hell is going on! This is just another case of men trying to make something as wonderful as sex into something better. Sex experts and macho-male types all brag about doing 'it' all night without premature ejaculation. These sexual practices allow men to fulfill their fantasies but that's exactly what it is, pure fantasy!

Why the engine fails

In truth every male has encountered premature ejaculation more than once. Making love to someone new brings about a lot of excitement that is very difficult to control leading to premature ejaculation. However, it is still possible for men to make love all night without resorting to Viagra or Taoist sexual practices. Every male knows that the tricky part of sex with a new partner is having her wait around long enough for round two. In round two men have more control of their sexual genitals and can make love all night without premature ejaculation. Men can blame eagerness, the jitters or nervousness for sprinting the first hundred yards in a mile 'lovemaking' race. But given a second chance he can easily catch up and make up the distance. In addition, having a long time partner helps men in their sexual control. That is why married men have better sexual experiences than single males.

Another reason for the male power failure has to do with the Taoist cardinal rule of 'Use it or Lose it'. OK, guys let me explain this rule as simply as I can, "If you don't have sex often, you will lose your ability to have sex!" Simple enough? Still not convinced? The Taoist rule of Use it of Lose it applies to everything, especially sex. If you don't use or practice a skill often enough you will lose your ability/skill or forget how to use it. For example, newlyweds make love often in the beginning of their lives together. After the newlywed period their lovemaking episodes are slowly reduced to, let's say once a week! As the years pass, they only make love once a month then only once every two months then finally never. Until the thought of making love to their partner seems absurd. There maybe a lot of reasons for this decline but one thing is for certain, when one doesn't have sex on a regular basis he/she loses everything that evolves around sex like their sex drive and ability to perform.

Whatever the reasons, the key to avoiding sexual decline or to anything for that matter is Balance. When you make love with the same person too often you will get bored quickly no matter how attractive your partner is. Making love with extreme frequency drains the individual of energy and increases longer periods of rest to recuperate. Making love too often also leads to boredom which then leads one to view love making as a household chore that is reluctantly done to maintain a happy home. The reason it is viewed as a chore is because couples only make love in only one area like in the bedroom. Gone are the days of making love in every corner of the house. The bedroom is comfortable, reliable and the most convenient place for having sex. This is unfortunate because this puts unintended pressure on couples to make love whenever they are in bed. So instead of just sleeping together they unconsciously think they should 'sleep together' on the bed. There are times when couples don't feel like making love and that is OK, but because they are in bed there is a silent obligation to do so which slowly turns into an unwanted errand.

According to Taoist sages, balance is the key to success in everything, especially when it comes to sex. So guys, when you honestly don't feel like making love or have the energy to do so then… DON'T! When you constantly force yourself to have sex every weekend because you think it's the Macho-thing to do it quickly loses it novelty and that's when you start losing your interest in sex.

Ask any Taoist sage and he'll tell you that having great sex all starts and ends with the mind. Remember that the mind and body are connected. Your body will respond to whatever you are thinking. If your mind isn't on sex then it is no use forcing the issue with a dose of Viagra. Aphrodisiacs, Viagra and other male sexual tonics work the other way around by bypassing the mind and affecting the body; the male genitals to be exact. This is a hopeless method of telling or forcing your mind to think of having sex. Males often think that the reason they are losing their sex drive is because the body is getting older. They are partly right because as one gets older some hormones are lost. However, their sex drive was lost in the mind first before it occurred in the body. The body was willing and able but the mind wasn't!

So how do you get your mind thinking of sex again? Simple, let it be! Your mind is so preoccupied with sorting out all your thoughts that the last thing it needs is you forcing it to think of sex! As Laozi stated, the natural tao of man is to act in a natural spontaneity way. In other words, since sex is one of the primary needs of man, your mind (if left alone) will naturally gravitate towards sex, therefore you will have authentic (as opposed to being coaxed into) thoughts of having sex. Once that happens your body will naturally follow!

Your body is always seeking a balance so don't be surprised that you are not genuinely thinking of sex all the time. Your mind and body will let you know when it wants sex NOT the other way around!

Sex, it's perfect the way it is!

As mentioned previously, separating orgasm and ejaculation to promote longer lovemaking and preventing premature ejaculation is like trying to separate Yin from Yang. I do agree with the Taoist sage concern that losing sperm without procreation will drain a man of his energy. I also agree that prolonging ejaculation will extend enjoyment of sex but I disagree with the idea of having an orgasm without ejaculation.

Premature ejaculation is normal but once a male has a steady partner he would learn to control it. Mankind is always trying to improve something that is natural to him and ends up screwing it up. Sex is a part of nature and one of the most pleasurable activities for mankind. Now just the thought of sex increases anxiety and nervousness amongst men because of their self-induced pressure to perform well which leads to frustration in the bedroom.

Part of the problem is that men (and women) had made having sex the pinnacle of all human experiences. So important is having sex in our society that everything men and women do in their lives, in the end thrives around finding the best partner for sex. We thrive for prestige, higher education, wealth and looking our best all to attract the opposite sex. We constantly fantasize about making love like we see in the movies and are disappointed when it doesn't fulfill our dreams. Men are always trying to prove themselves through their sexual prowlness. Men are no longer satisfied with having just one loving partner, now he dreams of two lovers at the same time or a fling with someone else. The simple act of sex has turned into a grand performance of leather gear and whips, all in an effort to make sex better. When it comes to sex mankind has strayed far from nature. Sex between a man and woman is a part of nature and is natural, orgies and leather whips are not. As always, mankind takes the simplest and most pleasurable activity in his life like sex and has made it complicated. He either over-indulgences or he too restrictive when it comes to sex. Examples of over-indulging of sex are orgies, having two partners at the same time, cheating on your partner, sex toys etc. Sex has become a carnival event for exhibitionists! A popularity contest to see how many partners one can have in a lifetime! A male uses sex as a symbol of his manhood. A female uses sex to represent how attractive she is. Gone are the days of two loving partners intimate in their own private moments. If mankind isn't over-indulging he is being too restrictive on sex. Religion uses sex to control the sexual behaviors of its followers. Strict guidelines must be followed by couples. For example, sex is only for procreation and between married couples, any sexual activity outside these guidelines is considered wrong.

If mankind would just find a balance between over-indulgence and restriction on sex, he wouldn't be so pressured and anxious and constantly looking over his shoulder when he has sex!

Disagreement

I disagree with the Taoist sexual practice of withholding ejaculation during sex. Withholding ejaculation, I believe is not in accordance with the Tao of Nature. Ejaculation is as natural as breathing. Withholding the release of sperm increases unnecessary tension within the male's genitals which might harm him. This is like sealing off a pipe that is going to burst and pushing the water back up against the pressure trying to push it out. There would be too much strain within the genitals. The so-called studies to prove this is possible are a little fishy at best. It seems like the typical male-ego thing to do, with every male trying to go one up on the next guy.

I believe that orgasm and ejaculation go hand in hand. There is no way around this natural function of the genitals during sexual intercourse. The Taoist sages were correct when they said sperm lost without the goal of procreation is a waste. For example a salmon fights hard to swim up the stream to mate and then soon dies after mating. It is said that the salmon has done its job and nature recognizes this and now it is time for the salmon to die. It is believed that after the salmon has wasted all his energy swimming up stream and mating, a chemical reaction is triggered within the salmon. This chemical reaction starts killing the salmon until it has no more life. Humans are in some ways like the salmon, males use up a lot of energy during sexual intercourse and die or age little after each ejaculation. The male gives up his Qi (sexual energy) for the purpose of passing it onto his children but if not then it is a waste, for sexual Qi energy is one of the elixir of life.

So what does sex have to do with aging?

Every time a male ejaculates he loses sexual Qi energy. Sexual Qi energy is one of the most powerful energies that a man can generate. Sexual Qi energy is sometimes called Life energy because it is in a sense, like the salmon, the salmon is essentially giving up its own live so that other generations shall live. After ejaculation the human body then has to take energy reserves from other parts of the body to reproduce more sperm. This is because reproducing sperm for procreation is the highest priority for the body next to keeping itself alive. As a result there is not enough energy (Qi) for other parts of the body to adequately maintain or repair themselves and therefore that part of the body ages.

While I do believe ejaculation is unavoidable; re-circulating the sexual Qi energy during ejaculation to renew the body is not. I'll explain my theory in three parts. The first part is that the male sperm has sexual Qi energy attached to it during ejaculation. Therefore the female is not only receiving the male sperm but his sexual Qi energy as well which is then passed on to the baby. The female sexual Qi energy is already in the egg; once the sperm enters the egg, the baby will have sexual Qi energy from both parents.

The second part is when the male has an orgasm and ejaculates. I do believe that he can circulate some of his sexual Qi energy back up the Micro Cosmic Orbit. Much of his sexual Qi energy will go with the sperm during ejaculation and the other bit will go back up the Micro Cosmic Orbit. Having some of his sexual Qi energy returned to him and re-circulating within the Micro Cosmic Orbit has many benefits. 1) His sexual Qi energy will be renew faster, 2) he will have some of his life energy back, 3) and he will recuperate faster and be sexually active in a shorter period of time and 4) sexual Qi energy will add years to his life; in a sense he is reborn.

In part three, re-circulating some sexual Qi energy back through the Micro Cosmic Orbit is not as easy as it sounds. During ejaculation the male must focus on drawing some of his sexual Qi energy up through the tailbone to start the circulation. This is done by pressing the tongue on the roof of the mouth to complete the Micro Cosmic Orbit and using Yi (Intention) to extract sexual Qi energy as it is leaving the body. It's like trying to detour cars in a speeding highway onto a narrow road. With practice (lots and lots of practice) more sexual Qi energy can be withdrawn back into the Micro Cosmic Orbit revitalizing the male.

Gaining energy from partner

In addition to retrieving sexual energy during ejaculation the male can also receive energy from his partner. This energy can be retrieved at anytime during lovemaking. There are only two places where the male can withdraw sexual Qi energy from his female partner. The first area is the vagina during intercourse but this is extremely difficult. During intercourse the male, (using Yi-intention) has to draw up sexual Qi energy from the female's vagina through his genitals to the back tailbone and up the Micro Cosmic Orbit. During this act he is also taking away his own sexual Qi energy from his genitals which may lead to a lost of erection. This, however, is where a female's sexual Qi energy is most abundant and powerful during lovemaking.

The second area is in the mouth or her breath. We take in most of our Qi through the nose or mouth so it is not surprising that we also breathe out Qi. A male may take in some of a female's sexual Qi energy through her mouth by breathing in when she exhales. This technique must be coordinated with a willing partner.

There is another cosmic orbit that is formed during intercourse between to lovers; I call this the Sexual Cosmic Orbit. The orbit starts at the mouth as both male and female connect their tongues together to complete one half of the cosmic orbit. The orbit then moves down the head and spine and then to tailbone and is connected through the genitals of the both male and female. This Taoist sexual Qi technique energies both lovers.

Simple-Minded!

All males are pretty simple minded creatures and like dogs in heat they only have one goal in nature. If they know that they can retrieve Qi energy through sexual encounters that will be the only outlet they will choose. All males only want do what is simple and most pleasurable. So if they can get Qi just by having sex they won't waste time performing the Three Treasures. A Taoist story to outline my point is in order here. 'A Taoist sage was teaching a young student about cultivating Qi for longevity. The Taoist sage started saying "You may gather Qi in many ways, through physical exercise, long hours of meditation, being honest and humble, through sex, practicing Qi Gong diligently, eating healthy and sleeping properly" The young student thought for a while and replied eagerly "Did you say SEX!" Now the simple minded student is only thinking of sex because it is the most simple and most pleasurable thing to do to gather Qi. "Forget about meditating for long hours and exercising!" thinks the young student. So for many years the young student forgets everything else his teacher has said and only wants sex to cultivate Qi for longevity. He fails miserably at lovemaking and cultivating Qi through sex. Years pass and now the young student is an old man. He has wasted his energy and has aged rapidly because of that. One day he passes by his former teacher walking along with a beautiful lady in his arm. To his amazement his teacher looks just as young and healthy as he did when he was teaching him. Stopping his former teacher, he asked "Teacher I was your unworthy student who only thought about cultivating Qi through sex and had not bothered to practice the Three Treasures. Now I am old, sick and tired. But you are still young and sexually active how is this so?" "You fool!" shouted back the Teacher. "I offered you a clear path to long life yet you took the narrow road to no where. Only by first cultivating Qi through the Three Treasures will you know how to cultivate sexual Qi energy!" with that the teacher left his former student to his life of misery.' So one shouldn't cultivate Qi from only one source when other ways are also needed. The secret to cultivating Qi and achieving long life is balance.

Time

Have the time?

What is time? The dictionary says that it is a marker that measures changes. But in reality there really is no such thing as time, just the concept of it. Our concept of time is one of the major obstacles that have held us thinking within what I call, the Box. The Box is the conventional way of thinking or a way of understanding things that everyone in society adheres to. When one accepts conventional thinking without question then one begins a lifelong journey of hindering their natural and original way of thinking and being controlled by outside influences. Time is only a concept invented by mankind to measure the changes he was observing. He may have begun measuring time using the stars then the changing of the seasons and now he uses complex mathematics to measure changes to a millionth of a second. Like a two-sided sword, the conception of time has aided mankind but at the same time has become an invisible barrier that has controlled his life.

Time has created deep rooted beliefs or assumptions of aging. As we watch our elders change as time passes we make conclusions that they are growing old. So when one is at a certain age, for example fifty years of age, there is assumption or image that society expects to see of that person. The time of fifty years of existence comes with its core beliefs or assumptions and expectations. If one doesn't fit within these assumptions there is disarray and or other explanations are considered to explain this defiant variable. For example, if ones biological age is fifty everyone expects that person to show the signs and symptoms of a fifty year old person. But supposing that person only looks half his age, say early to mid-twenties, this mismatch of information causes the mind to find some rational explanation. One explanation is that the person is lying or there may have been a mistake on his birth certificate. Even when the person finally accepts the situation, there is still exists some doubt. Author Deepak Chopra recites from his book, 'Ageless Mind, Timeless Body', the core belief that many have about time, "Time is seen as a prison that no one escapes; our bodies are biochemical machines that, like all machines, must run down".

So how do we escape from this prison of time? Laozi believed that any convention (such as language) that controlled or blocked spontaneous thinking (original thought, ones own personal way of viewing things) was wrong. Zhaungzi added that language is natural and that we should use these conventions only as a means of functioning (communicating) within our society but to avoid entrapment of its beliefs (words change our perspective of things). So we should not abandon the idea of time but use it to help us function within our society like getting to work on time or keeping a time schedule to get things done and so on. But we should not let our concept of time dominant on all aspects of our lives, especially aging.

As Einstein once said time is relative. Two minutes sitting on a hot stove may seem like forever to the person sitting on it. But two minutes talking to a beautiful girl seems like a short time for the guy chatting with her. So time is all in ones perspective which means we can control how we experience it.

I had chosen to publish this book just before I reached the age of fifty. To most people, fifty years of age represents the half way point of one's life; to me it represents the beginning. The first fifty I spent experiencing and enjoying my world, the next fifty I'll spend understanding it. For me the last twenty-three years, time has stood still. You could say I was too busy enjoying myself and experiencing new things that I lost all sense of time (all twenty-three years worth). I believe I experienced what Zhuangzi described as acquiring a unique skill that was conducive to being one with nature. I was so wrapped up or involved with my particular skill (cultivating the Three Treasures) that I have developed, that when performing it I was in a 'spontaneous flow'. My particular skill was preserving the Three Treasures in my own unique way. You might say I've been performing my unique skill in a spontaneous flow everyday for the last twenty-three years and still continuing to do so.

My mind wasn't trapped within the conventional way of looking at time which I believed helped me to maintain my youthfulness. In my opinion, time and growing old was only a conceptual idea and only existed within the realm of the human mind. I asked myself this question everyday, "If there was no such thing as time then why should I grow older just because another year has passed?" Over twenty years later and I'm still asking myself this same question with the same answer: If time doesn't exist then aging shouldn't exist either.

Many have heard of these concepts before from ancient sages or from men of great minds but still have not grasp the concept or embraced it. Just because you are reading this information now doesn't mean you will embrace its concept. In order to change your views these revolutionary concepts must be adopted into your core belief system. Once you fully accept that time is but a fragment of our imagination you will be reborn. This is because by freeing yourself from the prison of time, you realize that there are endless possibilities and eternal hope in your life. You are no longer trap by the old concept of time.

Man is the only animal that recognizes that he is aging. Man is the only animal that can change his biological functions at will by changing how his mind thinks. Therefore if the mind is free from the confines of time, the mind can then alter the body with new potentials!

The Chaos of Nature

So if I practiced the Three Treasures religiously I will never get sick and never die? Wrong! Even the ancient sages realize that physical immortality was limited (they, however, believed that you can achieve health and longevity many times higher than the maximum age the average person lives today e.g. 80 years). However, if one lived within nature the concept of obtaining a long, healthy life is within ones grasp. Most of the time nature is in perfect harmony and everything is as it should be but from time to time informalities do occur. We often call these informalities disasters or give them horrific names to label and describe them. This is because they do not fit in the normal way or pattern that we are accustomed to viewing nature. But in truth they are part of nature, they are the Chaos of Nature.

We tend to see things in nature as being linear, everything happening in linear time and in a standard and unchanging pattern. But we fail to see all the invisible variables that affect these patterns. For example, a dripping faucet seems to drip in a fixed pattern. Given that there is amble supply of water and that no one adjusts the tap, the faucet will drip the same way and land on the same area every time. However, we don't realize that at any given time the rhythm of the falling droplets and the area which it lands can change. This is because like everything else in nature there are a lot of hidden variables at work. Invisible to the naked eye every drop is formed differently, the pressure to squeeze out each droplet through the faucet changes constantly, the air particles around the sink and within the bathroom fluctuate every millisecond and numerous other invisible variables take place. In the bigger picture, there seems to be no change in the dripping faucet but a closer look shows quite the opposite. If you ever had some time to kill you can stare at a dripping faucet and notice that at times the dripping, which you thought was constant, all of a sudden skips a beat or drips randomly then returns to normal. This is the invisible chaos of nature at work.

Scientist wanted to see the nature of chaos at work and prepared an experiment to test it. They instructed a computer to draw a complex pattern over and over using a preprogrammed algorithm. They expected to see no change to the drawing of the pattern and left the computer running the same program over a period of time. To their amazement within a few hours the computer had somehow bypassed the program and drew random and bizarre patterns. The chaos lasted only for a few seconds and returned to drawing the same pattern. The scientists were baffled by this. According to their calculations the computer should have drawn the same pattern infinitely. The reason they couldn't understand it was because they failed to see or recognize that random invisible variables can occur anytime and anywhere. The nature of chaos is unpredictable, there is no point in trying to understand the indescribable, it is what it is!

Rare human diseases and deformities are also considered a chaos of nature. Most of us are fortunate live without these problems but it does occur in some of us. The human DNA does its job 99.9999% of the time, it's as close to perfection as we can get but it is not out of reach from the nature of chaos.

How does this concept work
within the human body?

Just because you preserve the Three Treasures doesn't mean you are preventing chaos of nature from happening to you. Chaos may occur in many different forms within the human body such as irregular heartbeats, loss of sight, tumors just to name a few. Irregular heartbeats are just like the leaky faucet, once in a hundred thousand beats the heart skips a beat. Or you may have inherited genes that will cause some informalities like cancer, immune dysfunction, baldness etc. some scientist view aging as a mini form of chaos taking place every moment within our bodies. Some cells for no reason simply die or malfunction. Even your brain's neuron synapses misfire once in while.

So what is the point of preserving the Three Treasures if chaos of nature will occur within our bodies anyways? Minimum chaos is actually needed to rebalance the body. For example, your stomach lining is destroyed and replaced on a regular basis. Why? Because a new lining is needed to absorb the acid within the stomach, if it didn't you would die. Another example is your skin cells. Old skin cells are destroyed so that new ones can take their place to better protect the skin from external forces. It is only the large scale chaos that occurs like heart attacks you have to worry about. Preserving the Three Treasures helps you keep 'most' of the body in harmony, chaos is inevitable but keeping it to a minimum is well within our ability. If you have a heredity disease then unfortunately you are stuck with the genes that trigger them. But this doesn't mean that you can't keep them at bay or even reduce their capability by preserving the Three Treasures. Many of the things that we associate with aging (e.g. heart attacks) are simply chaos of nature within our bodies waiting to happen if we don't look after ourselves. Preserving the 3T's will keep most of the chaos at bay and even minimize their effects and keep the rest of the body in perfect harmony.

In the same way anti-virus cells are produced to destroy foreign cells to protect the body, your body already performs the same thing to old, dead, damaged and diseased cells. Your body has the task of constantly renewing itself by removing dead, bad or damaged cells and replacing them with new ones. This job gets harder as we get older and as a result, our bodies can't function at the same level as when we were young. So we have to give our bodies, especially the immune system, a lending hand by increasing our Qi levels. When one increases and strengthens the body's Qi, the Qi along with the immune system will keep the body healthy, vigorous and strong.

.

Vaccines, Hormones

I was quite nervous when I received my Yellow Fever vaccination. I haven't visited a doctor since high school and that was at least thirty-one years ago. This isn't because I don't like doctors or there was a genuine fear of them. It was just that I never got sick or ill enough that required me to visit my doctor. I had dispensed with the yearly medical checkups because I have developed an innate insight to my own health and well-being.

But because I was going to South America it was mandatory that I receive my vaccination. The reason I was nervous was that I didn't like the idea of putting something foreign in my body. I always believed that living a healthy lifestyle and cultivating my Qi energy would strengthen my immune system to fight off any disease or sickness I would encounter in my life. My trust in my immune system was rewarded with never getting colds or illnesses since I can remember. This doesn't mean I won't get infected, or injured. What it means is that I have faith that my immune system was strong enough to deal with any foreign viruses quickly and that symptoms and discomforts would be minimal. My belief was that if you took medicine for simple discomforts like colds, headaches and aches and pains you are simply making your immune system weaker. The human body is one of the most complex and miraculous organism on earth, and the immune system plays a vital part of our survival. We simply don't give the immune system a chance to recognize and destroy foreign viruses on its own and in the end we make it weaker and dependent on external aid like man-made drugs. Staying healthy is the best prevention and best defense to fight illnesses. This motto has kept me healthy and active for most of my life.

That being said, I had a lot of questions for the doctor and nurse giving me my vaccination. I thought the vaccination consisted of medicine that would stay in my body and was only used if it encountered any unknown viruses. What the vaccination really is a mini version of Yellow Fever, a strain of the virus. Once injected it was to be detected by my body's defense mechanism which then creates anti-body cells that will destroy it.

This works the same way for other vaccinations such as Flu shots. There are shots for different types of diseases and all are actually little version of the bigger viruses. The theory is that these shots help the body create anti-body cells for each vaccination introduced into the body. The anti-virus cells that were created stay in the body only for a certain period of time before they die out and then you would need another shot. So you may have both anti-virus cells for Yellow Fever and anti-virus cells for the Flu and another set of anti-virus cells for something else all swimming around inside you at the same time.

Vaccinations force your body to create an anti-body it may or may not need. In theory, these anti-bodies die out after a few of years which is why there is an expiry date on your vaccination card. You may need to get vaccinated again in the future with a different or stronger strain of the virus. Have you ever wonder what happens to these anti-bodies if they don't die out. Every living thing has an innate urge to survive, a sense of self-preservation that kicks in; and these anti-bodies are no different. If these anti-bodies are not fending off a particular virus, they are like anything else that is alive and want to survive; therefore they may mutate and start feeding off other cells in the body which would lead to other complications.

Ever wonder why some people who got vaccinated for the flu and still get it anyways? Your doctor will even state that this vaccination is not a 100% prevention. One reason is that the strain of virus injected into you to force your body to produce anti-body cells is just a mini-version of the virus. The anti-bodies created from that strain were only prepared for a mini battle not a full blown war, if and when the person contacts the full version of the virus. Your anti-bodies were prepared to face the school bully but not the rest of his gang. But have you ever known of anyone who had the mumps or measles as a child catching it again? No! And that's because the body was given the chance to create real anti-bodies to fight off a full strain of the virus that caused either the mumps or measles. The main reason for the vaccine is so that the virus doesn't spread to other people. But the hidden reason is that no one wants to suffer through agonizing symptoms (body's reaction) and the recovery period (the body's anti-bodies vs. virus). People with mumps display swollen cheeks and individuals with measles have nasty red rashes all over their bodies that may leave scarring.

However, in both cases these individuals are protected from ever catching these viruses again because the body suffered through the symptoms and was smart enough to create real anti-bodies that were prepared to fight an army of viruses if it had to.

The second reason is that the viruses change constantly, so the strain injected into you may not be the same strain you come in contact with. Many of the old viruses are constantly developing new and stronger strains so the need to upgrade vaccinations is a must. This cycle of vaccination will never end. Nature is always reinventing herself and it has been doing this since the forming of the earth. In the long run nature will win unless man changes its way of thinking about illnesses and disease. The real problem is that mankind is fighting against nature and trying to control it instead of trying to understand and work with it. Man is a part of nature and the more he tries to separate himself from it the worst his status within nature becomes.

Taking hormones to replace depleted ones

Like vaccines, hormones are taken for various reasons. Hormone therapy may be used for people whose own body cannot create enough of it to sustain a healthy life or someone suffering from dwarfism or for other purposes like bodybuilding. Bodybuilders inject hormones to create bigger muscles. One use is a necessity (dwarfism) the other is for vanity (bodybuilding) but regardless of how they are applied they are still ejecting a foreign substance into the body. The body still recognizes this hormone as a foreign substance. In the short run, hormone therapy works wonders for restoring vigor, building muscles and increasing sexual functions. However, at the same time the body's immune system still wants to destroy this foreign substance. The body may do this by creating cancerous cells. That is why people on hormone therapy run the risk of developing cancer. If the body isn't producing cancerous cells it is then destroying other body parts in reaction to these foreign hormones. Individuals who take growth hormones (steroids) to build muscles and increase athletic performance or increase ones libido fail see the side effects during and even after they stopped using steroids. Hormone ejection works wonders at first because of the body's initial reaction to it. Just like taking a vaccination there are initial symptoms one might occur like a fever or headache. This is the body's reaction to the foreign substance as it builds anti-bodies to fight it. So the person taking steroids wants the body to react by creating bigger muscles (symptoms). Just like taking vaccines which may result in symptoms of headaches, a bodybuilder's symptoms (bigger muscles) are also short-lived and one has to keep taking hormones to maintain the results. Foreign hormones injected into the body are absorbed into the blood stream; they do not remain in the body for very long. Like vaccinations these foreign hormones are treated like foreign strains of viruses. The body will make anti-hormone cells that will search and destroy them. Frequent use of hormones is like frequent use of vaccines. Soon the body will create so much anti-hormone cells that the body starts destroying itself. Can you imagine vaccinating yourself every day? Sound insane doesn't it? But that is what one is doing when taking steroids/hormones on a regular basis.

Taking hormones increases your metabolism and ages you faster than you normally would. A teenager taking steroids will mature faster than his friends who are not taking it. This is because steroids force not only the muscles to grow bigger and faster; it also forces the entire body to grow and triggers an early maturity stage before the body is ready. Unfortunately because of steroids the teenager using it will also age much faster than his friends; even after discontinued use.

Instead of ejecting hormones, one should try to increase the hormone production system within ones own body first, instead of replacing it with a foreign substances. Both Taoist sexual practices and herbal medicines can increase ones hormone production system. Unfortunately these practices will aid in only producing normal amount of hormones needed for healthy body function, not the excessive amount needed for athletic high performance or for bodybuilding. But in the long run it is a safer and healthier method to increase hormone production within oneself, and that is Taoism's main goal; keeping you healthy and youthful till old age.

Values

Being materialistic

Give a man one million dollars in cash and by the end of the day he would have spent it all and worst, he'll be indebt. Give a man several cars and he'll find a reason for wanting another one. Give a man enough rope and he'll (... put in your own words!) Give him all the necessities of life and he still wants more. This is because he lives in a world that believes it can buy happiness, enlightenment and even love at discount prices. He thinks that these concepts are tangible items he can pick up at a department store on his way from work. He lives in a materialistic world driven to consume more than he will ever need. For an example, infants will only eat till their bellies were full; they instinctively know when to stop. Today as adolescents and adults they still keep on eating even when they are full. It's because society has conditioned them to do so.

Laozi has forever preached that humanity should only be interested in satisfying his primitive needs of food, water, sex, shelter and living in a clean environment. Once he has done this he would no longer wish or pursue unnatural desires. Unfortunately mankind is no longer satisfied with meeting his primitive needs and continues to seek more. Since leaving the Garden of Eden, mankind has been on an endless search to satisfy his unnatural desires such as materialistic goods.

For centuries mankind had simply followed the standards set by his society. From a Taoist point of view this is not the true nature of man, or the Tao of man (the true guiding way of man). In other words this is not how mankind was supposed to act. His priority should be to his primitive needs and be satisfied, not in spending most of his life of pursuing and consuming and acquiring selfish goods.

Language

The two great Taoist sages Laozi and Zhuangzi would argue that language and perception are some of the reasons humanity is so materialistic. They would point out that the use of language creates distinctions of things. For example once we know what is beautiful we automatically know what is ugly. If something is good the other must be bad and so on. By making distinctions we learn to be discriminating which leads to chronic dissatisfaction because now we only want what is considered the best as compared to the worst things for ourselves. We are no longer satisfied with what we have and are continuingly searching fruitlessly for the best clothes, the finest food and so on. According to Laozi, acquiring of such extravagant and sophistication is unnatural, it is an unnatural desire that has consequences. The Daode Jing or should I say Laozi, suggests that language creates social control that blocks our natural spontaneity and that we should avoid learning language. Many of the Chinese scholars of different philosophies joined the Laozi bandwagon to advocated abandoning language altogether. Language is defective they claimed. Since learning a language is knowledge, they said that we should abandon knowledge also. But Laozi was more concern about the knowledge that made distinctions of guiding behavior. Conventions (such as language) that were seen as a way of controlling people, distorting their natural desires and natural spontaneity should be abandoned. Language in this view only gives new unnatural desires for things they can distinguish.

Zhuangzi recognized that language is a convention that is natural and allows people to communicate. The problem is the perspective that people associate words with such as beautiful and ugly. Others may find what you consider beautiful as ugly. The critical step in any knowledge is, as Zhuangzi would say, an appreciation of other people's point of view. In this way, language won't distort or shape your natural behavior because you are open to appreciate a different interpretation. People should accept conventions for their own sake. Language is a useful convention that helps us communicate with others but that is all. So it is OK to conform for practical reasons but not from a conviction that raises prejudice or sets standards of living that everyone should live by.

So what does language have to do
with staying young?

The key here is listening to your own Tao or following your own path and not letting others or society control or block what you were meant to do. Language is a convention of humanity but the ancient Taoist sages observed flaws in its usage. They believed that language that controlled the actions of people should be avoided. For example, society considers you old because you're sixty-five and forces you to retire. You may not feel old but according to society when you reach that age you are useless.

You are forced into retirement when you are perfectly fit and healthy. From society's point of view, at sixty-five you are no longer able to contribute in the work force, you are supposed to be old and grey with a hunched back and a burden on society and so on. Language has so much power, that it changes everyone's perspective into one common theme. It changes your perspective until you start to believe in them and conform by getting older and growing grey hair and developing a hunched back. So always beware of what is communicated to you or what you hear. Language can affect your perspective of things and can even age you without you even knowing it. The way to combat the affects of language is to always think positive of yourself and have an open mind towards everything.

Our Primitive Needs

To the Taoist everything is connected. Following materialistic conventions like buying goods are OK when satisfying your primitive needs like eating when you are hungry. But consuming unnatural desires like vanity when you still have to eat or pay off the mortgage doesn't make much sense. Even though food doesn't last as long as a material item, it is a primary need and should be a priority. Satisfying our basic needs and not searching for unnatural desires keeps us young by freeing our minds and our thoughts to admire the beauty of our world and of ourselves. We can't do that if we're always thinking of buying excessive goods we don't need. We don't need materialistic things to tell or make us into something everyone could admire. We are perfect the way we are and who we are. We don't have to prove anything to anyone. We don't need to keep up with the Jones! When our primitive needs of food, water, sex and shelter are met we should be satisfied. People who have a sense of who they are and are happy show the most youthfulness. Youthfulness starts from the inside then goes out. When your mind is not preoccupied with material goods it has time to appreciate the more important things in life like family and friends, in other words it has time to be happy. A happy and well balanced person shows vitality and youthfulness in their outer appearance. Tranquility of mind and body leads to better health and longevity. Aging cannot affect a tranquil mind and a well nourished Qi body.

Returning to the child

Laozi would suggest to everyone that they 'return to the child'. Returning to the child would mean that to a child, everything is new and exciting. An adult may find a new television exciting but a child would be just as excited playing with the box it came in. So if everyone returned to the child they will find excitement in everything and start enjoying the things they already have. Returning to the child doesn't mean that all adults should act like children. They should, however, try to remember how they saw the world as a child and how everything was special. Infants and younger children are often used in Taoist analogies. This is because they represent the true nature of humanity in its purest form. Children are without hatred, greed, lust for power and discrimination. Taoist sages believed adults can regain much of their youthfulness through their children. Children are excited about everything, they are excited about life. Children remind us of what's really important in life. We should let children teach us how to stay young. As children they naturally follow a guide or path of nature but as they get older they follow an unnatural path created by their society.

Children would be considered what Taoist call a *'true person'*. For the Taoist, true people act authentically according to the ever-changing transformations of nature and the universe. For example children would laugh out loud at something they thought was funny regardless of where they were. They are not concern about being embarrassed or looking out of place. Their reaction is spontaneous and true and they act according to that moment (ever-changing transformation). In addition, children are true people because they do not deliberate their actions, but act from their inner most being. In all of us, there is an inner sense of the right thing to do and children act accordingly based on it. For the Taoist, a true person acts according to what they believe is right and not by society's standards. Unfortunately as children grow up their behavior and judgment are marred and shaped by their environment. By old age the same awareness that they displayed in childhood has been conditioned thousands of times until the mind becomes stiff and brittle which reflects in every cell of their body.

So what does Returning to the
Child have to do with aging?

The most youthful looking seniors are the ones who have not forgotten how to be a child. They are the ones who never let go of their inner child. This doesn't mean that they are not mature. On the contrary, growing up and being mature doesn't necessary mean letting go how you viewed the world as child. Creative people and geniuses have the most childlike attitudes towards their professions. Artists, scientists, musicians and creative people are gifted because they still see their world as they did when they were children. Forever excited about new creation and possibilities the child within them still lives. They depend on their childlike fantasies to see through the Box (conventional thinking) and envision all the possibilities.

Reversing Values

One of the most provoking statements within Laozi's Daode Jing is his idea of reversing of values. It was said that Laozi was against Confucius conventions. Confucius placed value on such things as being Yang, dominance, male, strong and aggressive. Laozi saw the value in its opposite such as Yin, submissive, female, weak and passive. Laozi figured that by learning the value of its opposite one would realize that there is another way of being, acting or looking at something. There are numerous stories in the Daode Jing (also called the Laozi, after its founder) about the value in reversing values. One such story was about an escort sent by the king to visit Laozi. The king thought Laozi was a wise man and wanted to offer him a high ranking position within the government. He sent his escort to find Laozi to offer him the position and return with an answer. When the escort located Laozi he was sitting by a stream looking at some pigs playing in the mud. The escort gave Laozi the king's offer to him. Laozi thought for a while then began telling a story to the escort. Laozi said "There was once a divine pig playing in the mud. A king wanted to honor this pig and had it slaughtered and put on a throne for all to admire". Laozi then asked the escort "Was the pig better off alive playing in the mud or dead on the throne?" The escort replied "Alive, of course" then Laozi answered "Tell the king that I, too, like the pig am happy just playing in the mud".

So what does Reversing Values
have anything to do with aging?

Everything! Laozi introduces the idea of reversing of values because he saw the value in its opposite. Instead of always seeing things from one perspective there is an equal worth from another perspective. Reversing of values opens peoples mind to the balance of nature in which they live in. Where there is Yang there is always Yin. Both are equal and in harmony with one another. In addition to helping people see the value in the opposite, reversing of values also makes them humble and appreciative of their life and the world around them. Seeing the value of opposites also helps people be more open to different interpretations of things. People are so conditioned by society to see things in only one way. Reversing values helps open new possibilities. For example an old person doesn't to have view themselves as worthless. There is value in old age. One doesn't have to associate feeble and senility with old age. One can also view old age as having wisdom and experience and knowledge. Reversing values opens our eyes to the opposite value and leads to creativeness, spur-of-the-moment actions and liveliness, things that are with associated with youth. Old people should not value youth more than experience for this leads to envy, discontent and stress and therefore accelerated aging. In seeing the value in themselves they are free of worry and the confines of old age that they have created for themselves. In the end, they are happier and more content which shows in their reverse youthful appearance.

Rarity

Materialistic things like diamonds are horded by people because of its rarity. Everyone wants them because there are so few. But if no one wanted them, diamonds would be worthless; therefore they only have value when someone else wants them. Gold is also a rarity. Clean drinking water in a modern city is cheap compared to gold. But on a remote island, fresh water is worth more than gold. So something is worthy depending on one's perspective. Just like a family heirloom is priceless to the immediate family, it may deem worthless to an antique dealer. We deem something worthy by its rarity and from our own perspective. From a Taoist point of view just because something is rare doesn't mean we necessary have to have it. If it doesn't satisfy our primitive needs its value is only secondary. Since rare things are only secondary you shouldn't place that much importance on them and quit wasting your time obtaining them.

So what does acquiring rare things have to do with aging?

There is an old Taoist saying that life is limited and the Great Tao is endless. One should not spend one's life (which is limited) trying to obtain the limitless – the Great Tao. An example would be knowledge. There is no way one could find the answers to everything in their lifetime so why bother? It would be a fruitless effort. How do we know our conventions are the correct ones? Better instead to enjoy the life you do have and abandon your fruitless search. In the same sense, you are only wasting your time trying acquiring rare things. This is because there are too many rare things which are limitless to acquire in ones lifetime (which is limited). In addition, rare things depend on one's perspective which changes often. Better to forget the rare things and spend your time preserving the Three Treasures to gain health, enlightenment, happiness and longevity in your limited lifetime.

A need to stand out from the crowd

A part of being materialistic is the need to stand out from the crowd and be noticed. Everyone likes being admired. Vanity is an indulgence after our primitive needs are satisfied. We like being part of a crowd but at the same time we like to stand out. We do this by acquiring rare things or materialistic things that give us the impression of importance, power and respect. Some people collect the rarest of wines, baseball cards or anything of rarity because they believe this makes them special too. Some develop a specialty trade or skill that would gain them popularity and importance. This too is an unnatural guide or path. People think they lose their identity, popularity and empowerment if they don't stand out amongst everyone else. But if they practiced Laozi's lesson about reversing values then they would understand why it is better to blend in with the crowd, go unnoticed and have a stable life. For example if someone thinks of you as strong claim you are weak. A strong person will eventually show weakness and will be criticized for it. Since nothing is expected of a weak person there is no pressure to live up to it. In addition, if a weak person shows strength from time to time, they are admired and praised. If a strong person did the same, it was expected and no one would notice any different. The lesson here is humility goes a long way!

Standing out from the crowd is easy, getting to the top is easy but staying there is a different story. Ones energy and resources are wasted trying to maintain whatever momentary status or empowerment they think they have gained being on top or standing out from the crowd. This popularity is fragile and will quickly disappear as fast as it occurred. This is what happens when you satisfy the Ego instead of satisfying your primitive needs. The stress of remaining on top, ages the body more quickly so it is better to live amongst the crowd anonymously, roll in the mud like Laozi and the pigs, and have a long and happy life.

OK, so how should we act?

From the book, "The Complete Idiot's Guide to Taoism", the authors hypothesized how Zhuangzi may have believed as the right Tao/Path to follow:

"Be open to new ways and flexible in incorporating them in your own way of life"

The world doesn't necessary have to evolve around your reality or interpretation of it. By being inflexible and rigid in your views you become closed minded. Others may have answers to any dilemma you may have but you won't know that if you shut out everyone else's opinions or interpretations. Don't forget that your interpretation and values are mostly shaped by society. Society's values and interpretations that have guided you aren't necessary the absolute correct way or path. Others living in a different country will have different values and interpretations which may be better. Instead of holding close to your values try being more acceptable of other interpretations and views and incorporate them into your life. We can never be sure that our perspectives are correct so it is better to have a variety of different perspectives to compare and make a judgment.

"Understand both the usefulness and limitations of conventions"

Zhuangzi understood that the conventions (such as language) allow us to communicate and coordinate our actions. Language however, should not affect our view and interpretations of our world. One way to avoid this is to learn several languages.

Each language carries different words for the same thing but with different meaning. This helps the individual be open-minded in terms of how to interpret his own language.

Remember, everything you have been told to do or taught are conventions of society. Mankind is limited and the conventions he creates are therefore limited. They are useful in getting things done but we really don't know if they are the 'absolute correct' ones to follow. We should just use them to be an effective member of society but be open to other views.

"Cultivate skill to the point of spontaneous flow"

Zhuangzi encourage everyone to master some Tao or a way or path of doing something in what Zhuangzi calls a Spontaneous Flow. In other words, be really good at something and immerse yourself into it. It could be something as grand as playing a musical instrument or something more intimate like making bowls, butchering or anything you enjoy so much that you feel an intimate connection with the world while doing it. Suppose you are a skilled wood carver and your mind was so wrapped up in a project you were doing, paying attention to every detail of your work. Every movement of your carving knife was precise, smooth and cut exactly where it should. Your mind was so focused on what you were doing that you didn't notice anything outside your workshop because you were in a spontaneous flow. So it really doesn't matter what job you do, just try to cultivate a skill within your job description and go with the flow. Zhuangzi often uses a butcher as a metaphor for cultivating skill. This is because butchering in ancient China was not a highly regarded position. Most of us may not have an occupation we enjoy doing but Zhuangzi wanted to emphasis that one can cultivate a skill to a point of spontaneous flow regardless of their job or what they were doing.

We should spend more time enjoying and doing the things we're good at and what gives us pleasure; by doing so it helps us connect with the world we live in, can you think of a better way to live your life?

Affirmatives

Y.A.T.H.E.S.

Young, Attractive, Tall, Healthy, Energetic and Strong. These are the affirmatives I repeat to myself when meditating. Affirmatives help you focus on the things you want in your life. As Zhaungzi would suggest language is a conventional tool that should be use to communicate. Language also has great hidden power. The language we use to refer to ourselves is very powerful for we literally create ourselves out of the very words we speak. Words program our subconscious minds into who we want to be and how we want to be seen. So think about words (affirmatives) of how you want to be and think about them often so that they become your dominant thoughts. To add more power to affirmatives say them out loud to yourself. When an affirmative is spoken instead of being thought of it carries more meaning and strength to your cause.

As I mentioned previously, when your mind is always thinking about something (your dominant thoughts), the body automatically tries to achieve whatever you are thinking about. For example, you may be thinking about losing weight, your body automatically burns more calories in order for you to achieve your goals. The more focus your mind is the more your body will react. The mind and body are one, what you think you are your body will become. And yes, this method of sending affirmatives while meditating does work on keeping you young through old age. Sending affirmatives while meditating is even stronger because when you send affirmatives to the mind when it is calm, it is in a better state to accept these affirmatives then trying to send affirmatives while on a busy bus going to work. Constantly reaffirming your goals is a must. This is because our mind always wants to absorb as much information on any given moment through our senses (touch, smell, sight, taste, hearing and thoughts). When much of what occupies our minds is our affirmatives then the mind will constantly tell the body to achieve these affirmatives.

Taoist sages were always focused on their goals and never let their minds wondered by incorporating their own affirmatives while preserving the Three Treasures.

Patterns

We all have developed patterns that we follow all the time in our lives. These patterns grew and matured as we did and are part of our characteristic make-up. These patterns could be positive or they can be negative. An example of a positive pattern is everything seems to go your way. Every time you enter a lottery you always win. You always seem to be in the right place at the right time. An example of a negative pattern in our lives is that you are constantly late for meetings, work, dates or any engagement.

Patterns are very difficult to change especially the negative ones. We obviously want to keep the positive ones and get rid of or change the negative ones. But changing a pattern that you have developed and nurtured into your subconscious is not easy. For example your negative pattern of always being late for everything. One day you accidentally leave early to a meeting and on the highway glance at your watch and see that you will arrive on time. You say to yourself "Hey, this can't be right. I'm going to arrive 10 minutes early" Your subconscious mind kicks in and says this is wrong and goes about changing the situation. You find the only road with heavy traffic or a tree to run into to stop yourself from being on time. Once you are successful in delaying your arrival time and are late once more, your subconscious mind says "Whew, that's better, everything is as it should be"

We begin to form behavioral patterns right from birth and they are persistent and firm. But we are not trapped in our patterns, though they are difficult to change they are not invincible. These patterns will change only when we change. You have to start by always thinking positive of yourself. Soon you will start creating more positive patterns and less negative ones.

Resistance is futile!

Said the Borg! The Borg is a space alien character in a sci-fi television series called Star Trek. The Borg captured other alien beings from other planets and turn into fellow Borgs. The Borg are mindless beings who are part alien and part machine, who have lost their will to resist their present state. But resistant is NOT futile! Remember all change is met with resistance but that doesn't mean we should give up like the Borg. For example, you start going on diet and the next thing you know you start getting invitations to dinners, parties, cookouts and anything involving food is at your door step.

In addition, you get comments from well-intended friends saying "You don't need to lose weight you look fine" and "its way too much work and effort, enjoy life to the fullest" But you have to persevere and keep focus on the change you want to happen. Be prepared for any resistance that will stand in your way. When you start practicing the Three Treasures to change your health, life or any pattern you wish to correct, remember you will be met with resistance. People in general would not understand what you are doing and will even try stop you and your motives will be questioned. They are actually challenging you to see if you are truly determined to do this. Once they see that you are determined and focused they will secretly cheer you on because they are admiring your tenacity. When you practice the Three Treasures you do it for yourself, nobody else. The only one you have to answer to is the person in the mirror. Practicing the Three Treasures is not an easy thing to do but it helps only having one person to answer to.

One cannot just start with the Three Treasures and not be changed in some ways by the Taoist philosophies that are deeply rooted in them. In addition, one cannot practice a Qi Gong form without a strong sense of direction, focus and Yi (intention). But the Three Treasures and Qi Gong can be practiced by anyone determined enough to change their pattern.

Waiting for things

Have you ever noticed that when you wait for things it never seems to arrive? When we wait for things it always takes a long time. But when you keep yourself busy doing other things then 'Bingo' it comes. The point is that we should get on with our lives and don't hold our breath for things to happen. Live for the moment! While you are waiting do something else, in this way you are detaching yourself from the end result. Therefore your happiness will not be determined by the end result but by how you are every moment of your life.

In my situation, while I practiced the Three Treasures diligently in my younger years, instead of waiting for the results which was looking and staying young, I went about doing others things that were of interest to me and that brought joy to my life. The reason it took me so long to see the end results was that I had involved myself with other activities that brought me happiness. I still diligently practiced the Three Treasures and I knew if I kept on checking for the big reward everyday since I started it would seem like it wasn't working and would never arrive. I kept a focused mind and strong will throughout and had faith my big reward will soon come. It wasn't long before I put the end result (my big reward) in the back of my mind and just carried on enjoying my life. Even if I didn't get the end results I was looking for through the Three Treasures I would not regret any moment of it. Practicing the Three Treasures filled a void that was sadly missing and guided me to live a carefree and joyous life. But to my surprise after twenty plus years of restoring and developing the Three Treasures I finally did get the end results I was looking for. The end results were right in front of me from day one and I didn't even see it. Like everyone else I was looking for a grand event which in my case, accumulated over time until I was able to see it. The Three Treasures worked from the first day I started and each and every day since then. The end result was only noticeable only after I compared how others have aged around me. I don't think I would have been successful if I just waited for the end results. In fact I would have been bored and would have given up on the whole idea of Youthful Immortality if I didn't enjoy my life as I waited for the big reward.

The Year of the Rat

The Rat (Shy, Smart & Determined)

I never really paid much attention to horoscopes but in my search to find an answer to why I have kept my youth I had to investigate all possibilities and connections. It wasn't until I seriously looked at the characteristics of the year I was born under the Chinese horoscope that I believe that I may have stumbled into something.

It shouldn't be that surprising I was born in the Year of the Rat. Under the Chinese calendar individuals who are born in the Year of the Rat are shy, smart and cunning. They also live for the moment and are survivors. In order to survive a Rat explores all his options. The Rat enjoys every moment of life because they are excited and curious about their world and like to explore and know more about it. Rats don't take sides in an argument and would like to remain neutral but is open to all interpretations. The Rat takes advantage of what nature has given him and doesn't seek more; it is happy with what it has. They are meek and non-aggressive but will be aggressive and strong when it has to. They are happy and care free and are only interested in satisfying their primitive needs of food, water, sex and a livable environment. Since they are very adaptive, they not only survive but can strive in any condition. Yup, that's me alright, a Rat and loving it.

If the biblical saying of "The Meek Shall Inherit the Earth" is true, then the future looks bright for Taoist adepts born in the Chinese Year of the Rat. All these characteristic traits fit into exactly how I would describe myself and how I react in real life. To me, the similarities are too close to be ignored.

So what does the Year of the Rat has to do with longevity?
As mentioned before, Rats not only survive they endure because they are creative, cunning and adaptive. The race to achieve immortality would surely be won by a person born under the Year of the Rat. And why not, the Rat was the first to enter Heavens Gate according to Chinese folktale. The folktale of how the Rat became the first animal to be allowed in Heavens Gate begins with a competition open to all animals big and small who have served mankind the most.

A race was arranged to see which animal would reach Heavens Gate first. Only the animals who reached the gate first would be let in. Now the Rat was thinking there was no way he was ever going beat any of the other animals in a race because he was too small. And there was no way anyone would even see him since he was so little. In addition, he offered no service to mankind. But the Rat was more cunning and clever than all the other animals. As all the animals raced towards Heavens Gate, the Rat asked the Ox "If you let me ride on top of your back, I'll show you a short cut to Heavens Gate? My legs are too small to walk the great distance" The Ox agreed and Rat went on top of the OX and both headed towards Heavens Gate. The Rat had chosen the Ox because he knew of all the animals on Earth, only the Ox had provided a great service to mankind and was also strong enough to walk the great distance to Heaven. Upon reaching Heavens Gate, the gatekeeper started opening the gates, and as the Ox proceeded the Rat suddenly ran and climbed up in front and onto the Ox's nose. "I'm the first!" proclaimed Rat. "Now you have to let me in!" The gatekeeper acknowledged and agreed that the Rat was indeed the first animal to reach Heaven's Gate.

Because of the Rats cleverness and determination to succeed against all odds he was let in. But now the Ox was upset that the Rat had tricked him but the gatekeeper seeing as how diligently the Ox had served mankind also let the Ox into Heaven's Gate. Other animals were let in as well but it was the meek little Rat that was the first to enter Heaven's Gate.

This is not to say that the person wishing to achieve immortality has a good chance if he was born under the Year of the Rat. He must, however, have the same determination and fortitude to continue the quest against all insurmountable odds. He must be like Water (a favorite element of the Taoist), adaptive, submissive and ever changing till the goal is reached. For example, all rivers lead to the ocean. Each river is met with many obstacles that block its path. Instead of trying to run over the obstacle the river simply submits and conforms and finds another path towards the ocean. So when trying to reach a goal be like the Rat or water and be determined, don't be deterred and always find new ways of reaching your goal.

The State of Non-Change

As one practices the Three Treasures diligently at a high level one will obtain, what I call the State of Non-Change. The State of Non-Change (SNC) is a state that you are in where Yin and Yang are in perfect harmony and you are one with Nature. You do not resist or try to change nature but flow effortlessly with it in your day-to-day activities. Your Yin and Yang energies are in perfect balance and old, disease or damaged cells are efficiently replaced with young, strong, vigorous, new cells, in other words everything is perfectly in sync. In the State of Non-Change one doesn't fear death but fully understands that without death there is no life.

I believe that when one reaches the State of Non-Change he/she is an Uncarved Block and every aspect of their lives functions within the Taoist principle of Wei Wu. What is meant by Uncarved Block or Uncarved Wood? The main principle of the Uncarved Block, or Uncarved Wood as it is otherwise known, is that things in their original simplicity or state contain their own power or natural beauty and function. When this simplicity is changed it is lost or ruined. This principle applies to people as well. Many try to change themselves from what they naturally are to fulfill unnatural desires such as power and envy. But in the end they simply lose themselves in the process. From the state of Uncarved Wood one can enjoy the simple, the natural and the plain. By being an Uncarved Wood one can see the beauty of nature in its own natural state and the Inner beauty within themselves.

When someone has reached the state of Non-Change they go along performing things in a Wei Wu fashion. Wei Wu is a Chinese term meaning literally 'Without Doing'. It is one of the main characteristic elements in ancient Taoism philosophy. 'Without Doing' also means 'Without Making' or 'Without Causing'. In other words without meddling, or combative or egotistic effort from mankind. To put it more clearly, Without Doing means not going against the nature of things or cleaver tampering to get what you want. The character Wei was created from the symbols of a clawing hand and a monkey, therefore the term Wei Wu would literally mean 'No Monkeying Around'

Water is often used as a metaphor to illustrate many Taoist ideas. Flowing water is very efficient because it follows an inert natural rhythm of things. All rivers and streams follow the path of nature and in the end flow into either lakes or oceans from whence they came. Each river and stream follows its own unique path without changing the natural laws of nature. Instead of trying to carve the most efficient route, it simply flows with nature and lets nature guide it. This means not forcing or trying to cut through a mountain if it's in the way but taking the easier and most effective route, like going around it. On the other hand, humanity's idea of efficiency is ramming through the most direct route while destroying everything in its path. Humanity's methods usually end up messing with the natural laws of nature. Zhuangzi wrote a short story outlining the powers of Wei Wu. In brief, the story goes something like this; fellow residents of a small village had witnessed an old man splashing about in a raging river. The old man was bopping in and out of the water, apparently trapped by the river. The residents rushed to aid the old man but by the time they reach the banks they noticed the old man was out of the water and singing along happily. The astonished residents asked how he survived. The old man replied that he grew up around this river and knows how to flow with the river. The old man said "I lose myself within the river; I go down with the river and come up with the river. I don't struggle with the rivers superior power!'"

Another individual in the same circumstance but without knowing about Wei Wu would struggle against the mighty river and fail and therefore drown. So the meaning behind this story is that when we work with our Inner Nature (one that we naturally have) and with the natural laws of nature we reach the state of Wei Wu. Just like the old man, we work with the natural order of things with minimal effort. Nature works within this principle and doesn't make mistakes or errors. For example, earthquakes are a natural order of nature. They are only perceived as mistakes from the limited mind of mankind. When you work within Wei Wu there is no stress, no struggle. The harder one struggle or tries, the harder it gets and it still doesn't work. Wei Wu doesn't try. Wei Wu doesn't ponder. Wei Wu just does. And when it does, it doesn't seem to do anything but things get done!

How long can one remain in
the state of Non-Change?

That depends! It depends on several things like your level of commitment to the practice of the Three Treasures; how balanced your Yin and Yang energies are on a day to day basis, how your outlook at life has changed or remained the same. Are you becoming an Uncarved Wood or are you slowly being sculptured and manipulated? Do you go about your daily life in a Wei Wu fashion or are you still struggling against nature? Immortality is as close or as far away as we wish it to be!

There are many things in this life that can tip us off the scale of a balanced life, it is up to each of us to recognize this and react appropriately according to our Inner Nature.

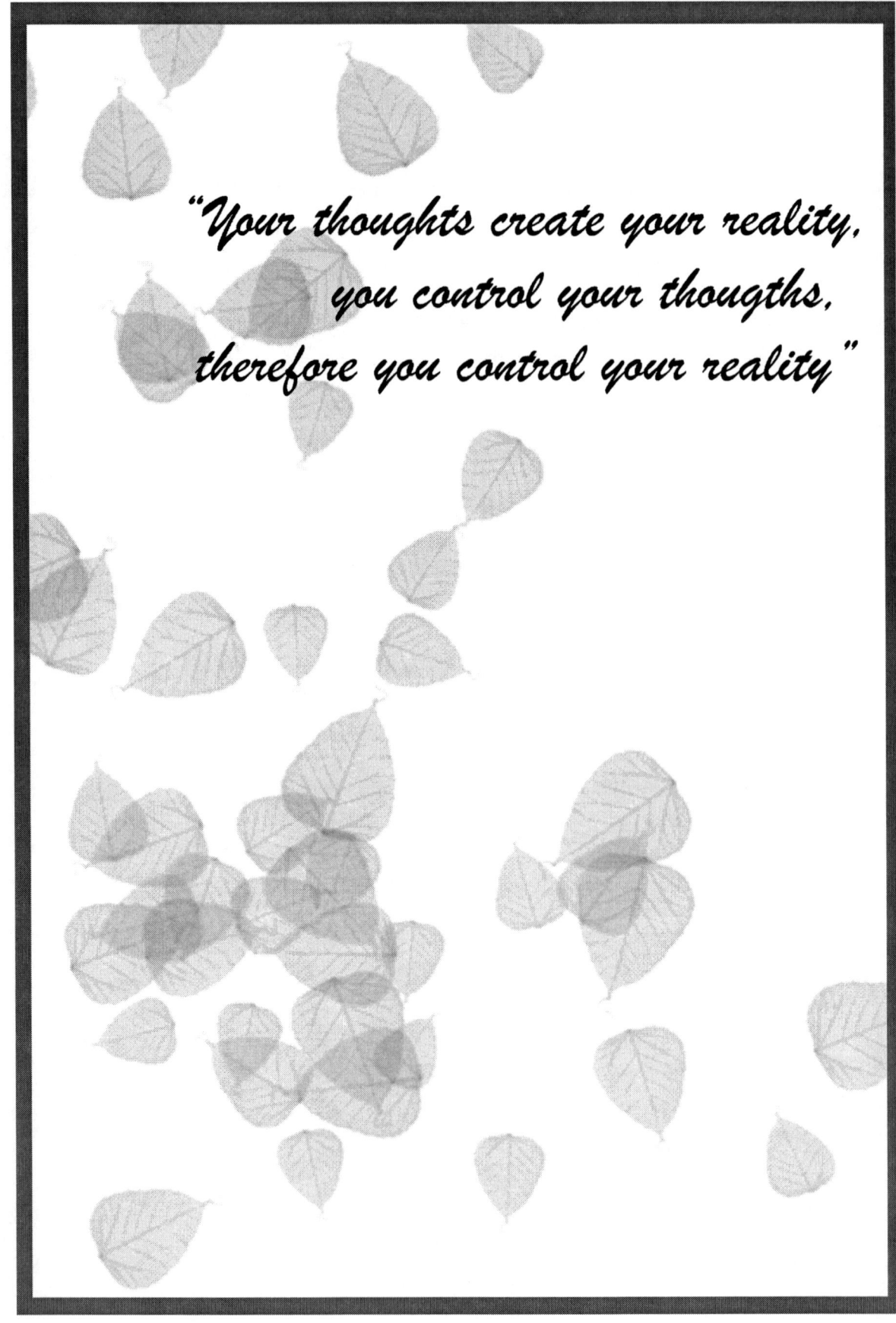

"*Your thoughts create your reality,
you control your thougths,
therefore you control your reality*"

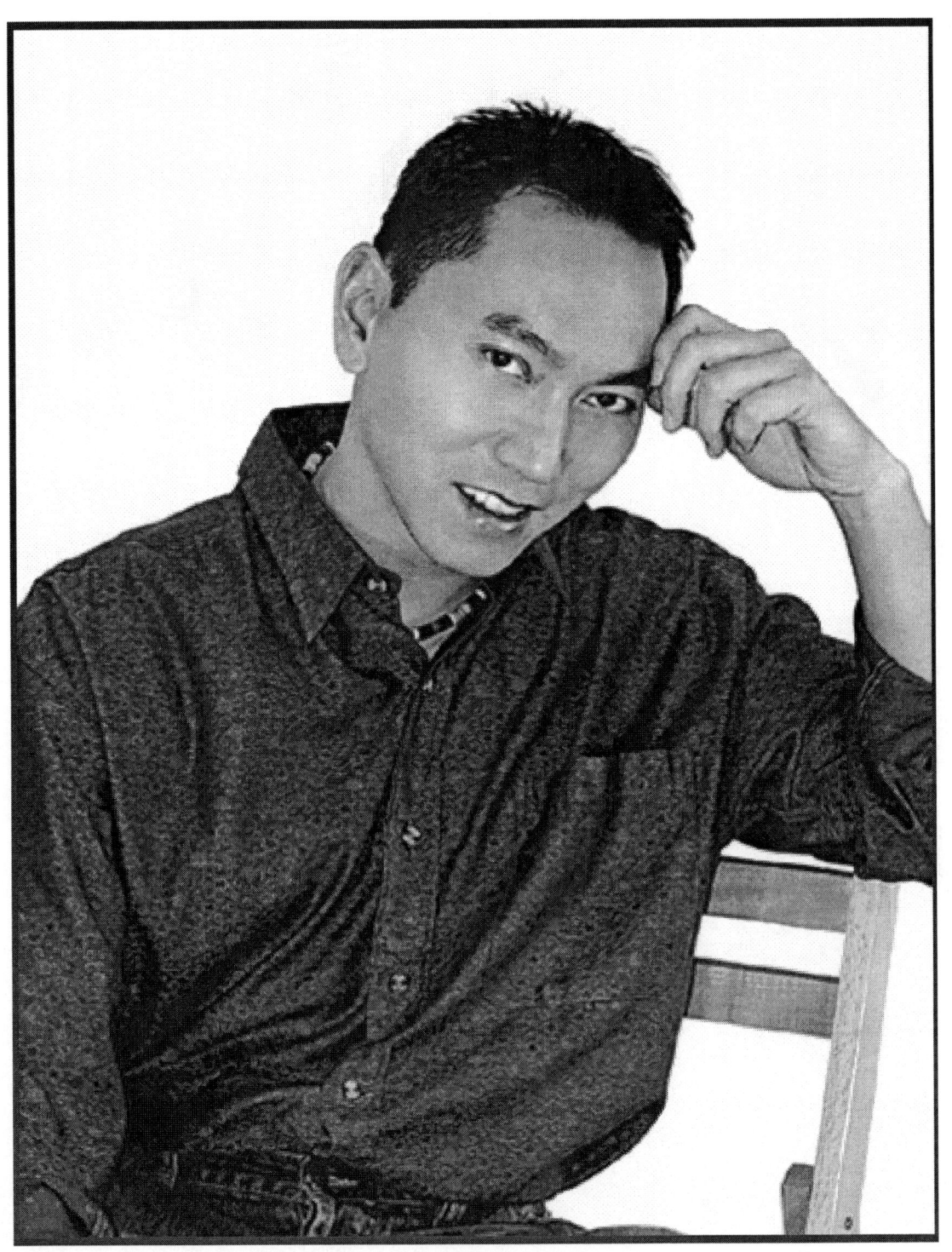

Norm Than at age 45

Final words

"An Enlightened Mind… is a Freed Mind" N.T

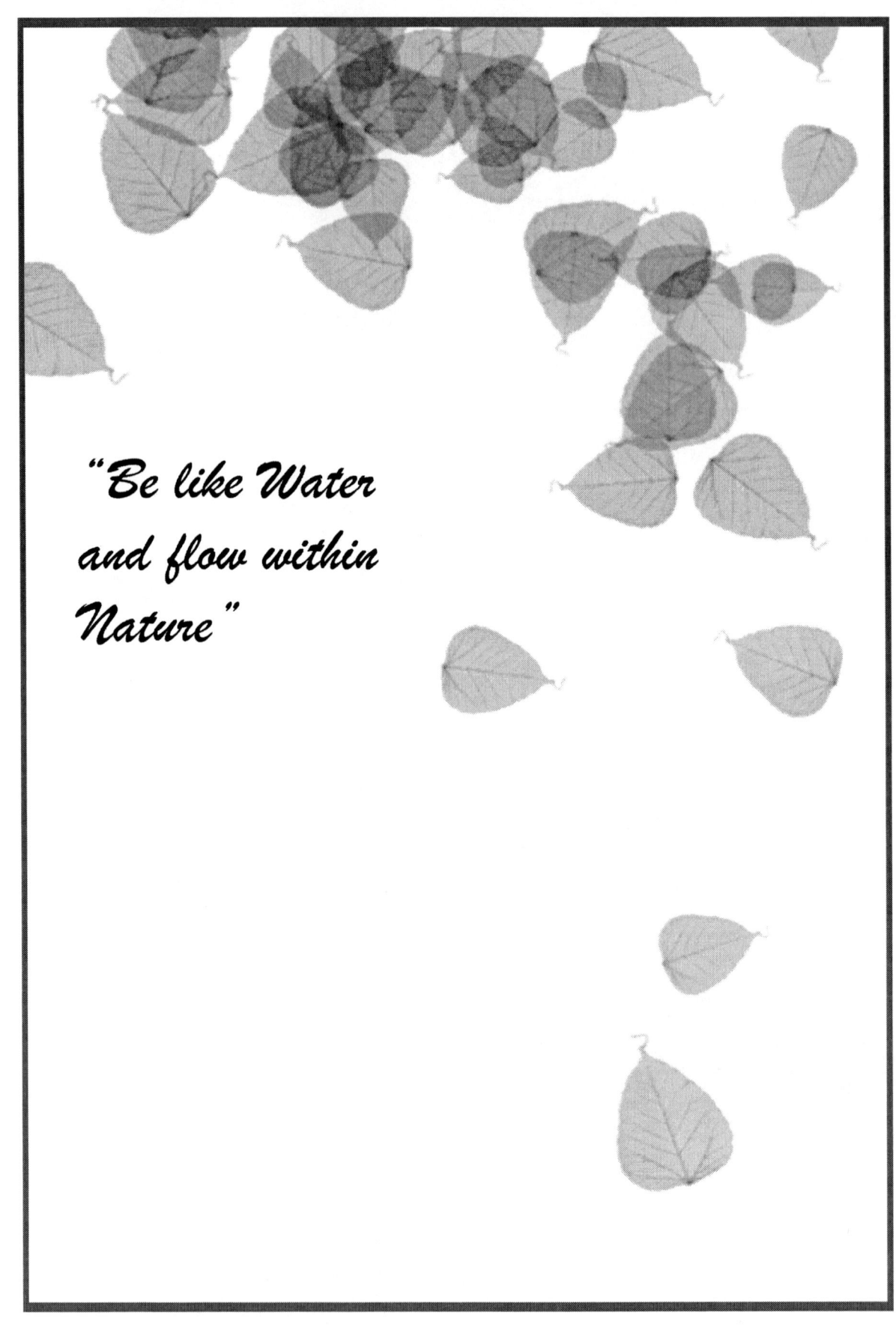

*"Be like Water
and flow within
Nature"*

Final Words

Summary

So here we are at the final chapter of my book. Together we have explored ancient Taoism and its realm of possibilities for achieving immortality. What have you learned about me, about my life, about the Three Treasures and more importantly about yourself? Do you have a better understanding of immortality from a Taoist point of view? Did I make you stand up and say 'Aha, I get it!' Let me take a moment to review some important points and include some more Taoist secret wisdom upon you just to make sure you got... IT!

Youthful Immortality-
Why most of us will not achieve it!

Understanding and acknowledging your own weakness is half the battle in any war. In preparation for your eternal quest you must be aware of potential hazards along the way. Some of them you will recognize, most of them you will not see coming until it is too late. The most humble, open-minded, diligent and most determined will succeed. Many will venture on the path to Youthful Immortality with few ever achieving their goals. For those who have accomplished something special, the road to Youthful Immortality was a pleasurable and spiritually uplifting experience. For those who found it difficult or have failed it was a perilous journey, filled with self-made barriers. In other words, they were their own worst enemy. These individuals did not grasp the concepts of Taoist immortality. For example, they did not understand the idea of living within nature or the working of wei wu. Nor did they did not have the right frame of mind, perspective and open-mindedness to recognize their own faults and adapt accordingly. In other words, these individuals may have been too materialistic and chased after the illusionary big reward instead of enjoying the view along the way. They may have been closed-minded towards their Inner Nature and did not trust in their own abilities but instead relied on others to guide them. However, the journey to immortality is a long one and often one will be confused and lost wondering along the way at times in their lives.

When we are on the right path to achieving Youthful Immortality there is a personal comfort zone we adhere to. In your comfort zone you find yourself being carefree and easy-going. When you start feeling uncomfortable, that is a sure sign that you are heading off the path. The simplest way to correct this problem and get back on the path is to first recognize this occurrence. Most often than not, these occurrences are not the result of external forces (things you can't control e.g. weather, earthquakes) but internal forces (things you can control e.g. your perception, being materialistic).

Being Aware Internally

As you read some of the Taoist philosophical concepts I have outlined, did you stop and say to yourself "I've experienced this before!" or "Oh, that was Wei Wu!" If you answered yes, it comes as no surprise because over the centuries Taoist concepts represent the Inner Nature of humanity and has interwoven itself in many ways into most religions and philosophies worldwide. So one may still innately experience and be aware of their Inner Nature, regardless of their religion and ideologies.

Not a Taoist, Not a problem!

The point is you don't necessary you have to be Taoist to be successful in practicing the Three Treasures. In fact we are all Taoist because we are all part of nature. Each and every one of us has experienced or followed some form of Taoist ideology in our lives without even realizing it. We experienced our Inner Nature at times without even trying and that's the secret to it all; and that's also our problem, we try too hard! We can only experience our Inner Nature when we don't think about trivia things that occupy our minds or when we don't try and struggle against nature. When the mind is empty and is not resisting, it will naturally return to its Inner Nature.

Personally, I was instinctively drawn to Taoism because it represented my true Inner Nature. Its philosophies on nature, society and the understanding of humanity and our world mirrored my own. I was following the footsteps of the ancient Taoist sages before I even knew what Taoism was. Taoism didn't guide me but offered the tools to guide myself.

Live within nature

In order for you to understand the what, why, where and when questions as you practice the Three Treasures, you should at least have a minimum understanding of Taoism.

The overall goal of Taoism is for all of us to live with nature and not separate ourselves from it. A core Taoist concept is that humanity by its own nature is good and happy and should live healthy and long lives. Within Taoism there are many paths to longevity with many different ideologies to what immortality is. However, there is one central idea and that is Youthful Immortality. The Taoist tradition of a Youthful Immortal is someone who, while still young, has discovered the secrets of life. The result is a long life of youthful appearance, outlook and energy. The Taoist Three Treasures (along with many other methods) has evolved over centuries to obtain the goal of Youthful Immortality.

For centuries in China, many Taoist sages have enjoyed long lives while the rest of their countrymen only lived a short time. The ancient Taoist practice of longevity was at first a guarded secret between student and master. But soon these practices were made available to their fellow countrymen. Many have taken up the practice and lived long lives but still many more have not.

The same problems that hinder many in ancient China from achieving Youthful Immortality are the same ones today the world over. These same problems in the past and today are not real problems at all, they are either imaginative or man-made. Our society creates our unnatural desires and controls our perspectives which in the end, stands in our way of understanding or listening to our Inner Nature and following the teachings of the ancient sages.

Ancient and contemporary societies have always thought to take the quickest and easiest route to achieving things and immortality is no exception. Our Egotistical Desires try and force youthful features through cosmetics, plastic surgery, rigorous diets and exercises. Our Cleverness tries to devise contraptions or magical potions or pills. Our Knowledge is too busy trying to figure out why we can't all live to be Youthful Immortals. But our Ego, Cleverness and Knowledge are limited. The only way is to Do Without Doing (Wu Wei Wu). This does not mean forgetting practicing the Three Treasures and being lazy and waiting for things to happen. What Wu Wei Wu means is that we should stop obeying our unnatural desires and depending on our limited Ego, Cleverness and Knowledge to achieve what will naturally occur. When we refuse to let our unnatural desires control us and realize our own limits we start listening to our Inner Nature which will naturally guide us.

Taoist practices are based on a deep connection and awareness of nature, for nothing is forced or cleverly devised to reproduce nature. The Taoist simply went with the flow of nature, since nature doesn't make mistakes they couldn't go wrong.

Great Reward

Our materialistic world believes that there is a great reward waiting for us somewhere and we have to work like crazy to get it. The great reward is always just out of our reach so we keep frantically going on hoping to obtain it. A way of life that keeps dangling a carrot in front of us with no hope of ever getting it is a wasted life. This makes it difficult for us to be Happy and Good which the Taoist believe is in our nature.

Once the big reward is reached, for example a promotion at work, all of a sudden the reward didn't seem that big of a deal. Only temporary satisfied we soon find ourselves chasing after another promotion or what we think is a bigger reward. The big reward may be in business, religion, athletic accomplishment or whatever, but the sad fact is it does not quench the never ending search for something better. We are too busy thinking in terms of fighting and overcoming believing we are making progress towards that reward. But real progress involves changing from within, unfortunately that is something people searching for the big reward are unwilling to do.

Your perspective on things

The reason it took me over twenty-three years to realize my big reward (remaining young in appearance) was because simply I wasn't looking for it. One thing I've learned over the years practicing the Three Treasures is that the rewards are instant. But in order to be successful you must cultivate your Qi everyday and live a balanced life. As I mentioned earlier, a balanced life can easy be skewed. For example, one day you may lose your loved ones in a tragic car accident or are financially ruin through the stock market or face other circumstances that throw you off your balanced lifestyle. Everyone experiences similar events but not every suffers the same, Why? That is because we can choose not to. The key is your own perspective on these events and not the events themselves which happens to all of us. How you perceive the events that happen in your life will determine your reaction, recovery and how well you will go on with your life.

My own tragedy

Like everyone else I have also experienced tragedy of both personal and financial loses. The death of mother and the lost my life saving in investments put tremendous strain on me emotionally. When my mother had pasted away I grieved for her. At that time I was working as a computer systems manager for an advertising company. My main job was maintenance of the computer system and the other was writing computer programs. This position was very demanding and took a lot of my private time but I enjoyed the work. News of my mother's death reached the office and I was allowed the customary time off to grief. During this time we buried my mother and got our family affairs in order. For three days my heart was filled with sorrow until I said 'Enough is enough' and headed back to work a week and a half before I was scheduled to come back.

Everyone in the office was surprised to see me back at work and in good spirits. Confused co-workers asked why I was back so soon and in my usual cheerful mood. I didn't bother trying to explain about my own Taoist views on death to them because I knew it would only confuse things. I simply said 'She's in a better place now and I have to start my life without her' In Taoism, death is perceived as a gateway to where we all began. Death is just another change in the flow of the Great Tao. I was sad at first but understood that she simply returned to what the Taoist termed Nothingness. From Nothingness everything is created. Another name for this is the Great Void. So my mother is actually back home, where she belongs and where we all will return, so why should I stay sad in this lifetime?

My own tragedy reminded me of a famous Taoist story about the pasting of Laozi's wife. Laozi was sad when his wife died. A few days afterwards a friend of Laozi's came to visit him to see how he was doing. To his astonishment he saw Laozi happily playing his favorite musical instrument. His friend was annoyed at Laozi for not following the customary rite of mourning (which was three weeks) of his wife's death. But Laozi said he was upset at first but realized that she simply had returned to where all life has begun. She had a good life and served her purpose here on earth so it was just her time to leave. The reaction of Laozi's friend, were similar to that of my co-workers and relatives at my mothers funeral. All my relatives expected to see me sad, which I was, and wail and cry uncontrollably which I did not. You see, many Asians are influenced by Confucius rites of moral conduct. The Confucius rite of proper mourning required living family members of the deceased to dress in white attire and show others how sad they were. To me this is simply putting on airs or a show for everyone else to prove how much I loved my mother. I loved my mother dearly and I didn't need to prove it to anyone.

When I lost my life savings during the brief recession followed by the high- tech market bust, I didn't fret like my friends. Sure I had bills to pay like everyone else who lost their money but I saw this as a lesson learned and went on with my life. It wasn't that I didn't care, it was just that I already had the things that were more important me like my health, family and friends. In my view I only lost what I considered was secondary in my life. My money could be replaced but my health, family and friends were priceless. I had the rest of my life to live and I'll be darn if I was going to let this one financial downfall ruin it. 'Stop and lick your wounds and learn from your mistakes and then get on with your life'… that's motto! Unfortunately, there are many who had lost their life savings who found it hard to go on. Their perception of their situation was worst than what it is really was. The situation will change as soon as we change our perception and reaction to it and not the other way around!

Rich or poor, we all suffer

The reason I brought up the topic of personal and financial loses in life is that we ALL experience these types of setbacks but NOT all of us suffer for the rest of our lives. Suffering is based on how we perceive things. These perceptions of ours have evolved since childhood and are deeply rooted but we CAN change them for the better. When you are practicing the Three Treasures, don't forget that you are going to be practicing it for a LIFETIME. Your path to success is aided by a healthy and positive perception of how you see events happening to you and how you perceive your progress of the Three Treasures. Remember, the mind and the body is connected. If your mind perceives something as hopeless (for example, the practicing of the 3T's) then your body will respond (aging quickly) to reflect what you are thinking. If you constantly let little events bother, unsettle or frighten you then your mind is in no shape to be practicing the Three Treasures. Same as if you constantly perceive small problems as big ones then your mind is already full of negative thoughts waiting for any excuse to set them free.

A journey of a thousand miles not only begins with single step but also with the right frame of mind. The practice of the Three Treasures should not be taken lightly. The rewards are infinite but the journey is long and difficult with many pitfalls. A weak mind filled with self doubt will be thrown off the path easily. But a strong and open mind filled with a positive outlook will succeed. Many will try the Three Treasures like they do any other exercise program. And like any program for your health it is a lifetime commitment. One can increase their chances of success with a healthy, positive attitude and a full tank of determination.

Instant gratification

If you find yourself skipping opportunities to practice one of the Three Treasures and or generally losing interest, it is because you are conditioned to seek instant gratification. For example, most people give up exercising not because it is too difficult but because they expect to see an improvement quickly. When they don't (which is a majority of the cases) they quit and think it's a waste of time. That is why I stressed the importance of having a strong Yi (intention) or will or whatever you like to call it. Your mind is always checking your thoughts, and if you're thinking of giving up then your body will react appropriately. Believe that the Three Treasures are working and it will reflect on your well being and in your youthfulness.

Another good quality to have besides a strong Yi is Patience. Patience is truly a virtue. When performing the Three Treasures, patience is a great asset. Not many of us have patience. Everyone is in such a great rush. We are in a hurry to get to work, to get things done, to have lunch, to get back home, to make dinner, to sleep and then in a hurry to start the whole thing over again the next day. We are even in a hurry to sleep which results in restless nights. In the end we are actually in a hurry to… save time! The funny thing is you can never save time you can only spend it. And we are even too busy to spend the time we hurried to save!

Nothing Doing or Doing Nothing

For many of us time is a precious commodity that should not be wasted doing NOTHING. So we purposely fill up our schedules with things we have no time for in the first place which means we place ourselves in a position to rush things just to get them done. But the Taoist saw great value in NOTHING. To the Taoist nothing is SOMETHING. The Taoist term the Great Void can be translated as the Great Nothing. In nothing, there is no beginning or end… it just is. Let me explain the term Nothing with an example. Has anyone asked you what you were doing? And you replied 'Nothing' But in fact you were actually busy working on a something, right? Have you ever truly done nothing? Not like being on a vacation doing nothing. When you are on vacation you are actually busy filling up your day with fun activities to do and that is doing something. And lounging around the beach getting a tan doesn't count either because you are still doing something (trying to get tanned). What I mean by doing nothing is that there was no goal or end result that was expected from it, there was no pressure, there was no destination point and there was nothing waiting for you at the end of it! If you ever truly did nothing did you notice how clear you mind was all of a sudden. For example have you ever wanted to remember something but just couldn't. And then you took a break to relax and did nothing and then BOOM what you wanted to remember comes into your mind? When a mind is freed from thinking of solutions, problem solving, expectations, dead lines it becomes empty and things become clearer. A freed mind is an empty mind, and it all begins by doing nothing. A Taoist sage will tell you that an empty mind can see what is front of it whereas an overstuffed mind can't! Remember in Star Wars, Luke was always told 'Empty your mind', because his thoughts where always in the past or in the future never in the present. And it was only by emptying his mind that he was able to understand the Force. The more filled or stuffed up your mind is, the less you hear with your own ears and see with your own eyes and the further you are from your Inner Nature. There is power in a clear mind which can be attained by anyone who can appreciate the value of Nothing.

Beware of False Masters!

As I previously mentioned, I am not too fond of what I call 'False Masters'. But as you progress in your training of the Three Treasures you should be open-minded to guidance from others. Unfortunately, there are many 'false masters' claiming this or that and with acts filled with smoke and mirrors. False masters seek the uneducated, gullible and foolhardy. Would you buy hair tonic from a bald person? No! Then why would you let an old man teach you the Three Treasures to staying young? Remember, 'A Tao that is constant is not the eternal Tao', use others only as guides, you are the only true master of your Qi.

I spent the first twenty-three years of my life perfecting the Taoist Three Treasures and spent the next twenty-three searching for the 'True Master' to show me the way to immortality. It wasn't until I gave up my quest did I uncovered my own revelation. Though my search ended in failure, through my journey I learned the two most important lessons in my life. And those lessons were 1) it is not the big reward at the end of the road that gives us the most pleasure it is the journey along the way and 2) we all have the determination, passion and power to achieve anything within us, all we have to do is believe in ourselves.

Even as I searched for the 'True Master', I diligently practiced my version of the Three Treasures to perfect my already high level of proficiency. The Three Treasures has become an important part of who I am. I found pleasure and sense of serenity whenever I performed the Three Treasures. In the end, it didn't matter if I found this 'True Master' or not, I was enjoying the journey more than the anticipation of the big reward. And through my enjoyment I discovered my own power and abilities and a stronger belief in myself.

The first lesson here is that reaching the goal or big reward is not as fun as proceeding towards it. The second lesson is that when one truly enjoys what they are doing they gain confidence through their own abilities and learns to appreciate their rewards along the way. Let's take the celebration of Christmas for example. Once all the presents have been opened and admired it isn't much fun anymore, is it? It was more fun thinking of the perfect gift for that someone special or the anticipation of what you hope you were going to get. But it was most fun remembering and participating in the real meaning behind what Christmas was all about; and that was being kind and opening our hearts to our fellow man. But why can't the spirit of Christmas occur in each of us 364 days every year instead of just one? If we add up all the big rewards (presents, promotions, good job appraisals etc.) in our life what we find is that they really don't add up to much. But if you also add up the spaces (the time of pure enjoyment working towards the reward) in between the rewards than we would have… EVERYTHING!

The Truth

The reason I talked about things like big reward, being materialistic, rarity, our beliefs etc. is that they are all illusionary yet they have such power and control over our lives. These are the things that keep us from living within nature and listening to our Inner Nature. So by putting little value on them we proceed to create minimum anxiety, stress, conflict and false expectations for ourselves. In the end, we begin to promote an efficient use of our mental and physical energies which will result in ease of mind and body functioning correlating directly to aging well. Therefore the more you naturally exist in the flow of nature the less wear and tear on your body and the less you age.

So be Good and Happy as nature intended while following the path to Youthful Immortality!